Detoxify Your Lifestyle

By
Dr. Nick Caras

Your New Lifestyle Starts Today

Dedicated to Mom and Dad for
all your unconditional love and support...

Lifestyle Habits

Lifestyle Habit 1. *Right Frame of Mind* – A time for Change
- Detox Quiz – Motivation
- Which Life Would You Choose at Eighty Years Old?
- Start Detoxifying your Lifestyle Now – Motivation

Lifestyle Habit 2. *Fats* – Which Ones Were We Meant to Eat?
- Detox Quiz – Fats
- Types of Fats
- What can high omega-3 foods do for you?
- Specific Conditions Fish Oil Supplementation will improve
- How to get essential omega-3 fats in your diet
- Start Detoxifying your Lifestyle Now – Fats

Lifestyle Habit 3. *Sugars*
- Think twice the next time you put sugar into your bloodstream
- Detox Quiz – Sugar addiction scale
- Start Detoxifying your Lifestyle Now – Sugars

Lifestyle Habit 4. *Your Gut and Bacteria*
– Good vs. Bad
- Detox Quiz – Bacteria and your digestive tract
- What our friendly bugs do for us.
- Probiotic Supplementation
- Start Detoxifying your Lifestyle Now – Our Gut

Lifestyle Habit 5. *Raw Foods and Greens*
- Detox Quiz – Raw foods and greens.
- Most and Least Pesticide treated foods.
- Most Common Genetically Modified (GMO) Foods
- Superfoods
- Start Detoxifying your Lifestyle Now – Foods

Lifestyle Habit 6. *Cleaning out Your Kitchen*
- Herb and Spice health benefit chart
- Start Detoxifying your Lifestyle Now – Kitchen Clean-up

Lifestyle Habit 1
Right Frame of Mind – A Time for Change

So why are you reading this book right now? What was your motivating factor to purchase this book out of all the thousands of books at the bookstore? Was it because you had a recent health scare, or someone close to you did and you finally decided to get off your butt and take control of your own health? Maybe you finally decided to jump on the wellness revolution bandwagon like so many others already have. Was it because your husband or wife hinted that you won't be here much longer if you keep living the lifestyle that you are accustomed to? A lot of us already live a very healthy lifestyle, and this might just be another tool to help keep us focused with our health and longevity in mind. Maybe your last yearly physical wasn't a positive experience. Maybe you are sick of that tire around your stomach, or maybe you are finally sick of feeling like crap every morning when you get out of bed. No matter where your current health is, good or bad, this book will take you on a journey to leading a much healthier, happier life. Whatever your motivation, I want to personally congratulate you for taking the first step toward the rest of your life. This book is full of information that will help you live the best life possible and enjoy the many fruits that life has to offer.

One of the major points continually stressed throughout *Detoxify Your Lifestyle* is to get back to the lifestyle of our ancestors. Don't worry just yet; I am not going to tell you to be a cave-dwelling, buffalo-hunting nomad, but we do need to get back to some of the original wellness habits that our ancestors practiced. Of course, there was no such thing as "wellness" back then; it was just a way of life. There is no doubt in my mind that we can all have that same way of life in today's hustle-and-bustle twenty-first century. This book will show you how to do just that. Throughout the book you will be reintroduced to how our ancestors ate, exercised, cooked, and relaxed. You will also be informed about how to incorporate these wellness habits in today's lifestyle. It is actually a lot simpler than you may think. There is a reason why we are a very unhealthy society as a whole, and by simply implementing some of the simple changes you will learn throughout this book and getting back to your roots, you can ensure the best life possible.

One thing that I can guarantee right at the start is that this process is not going to be easy. Why is change so hard? It is so hard because you are most likely changing something that you really enjoy, and this is why it is an addictive behavior in the first place. You have lived your "unhealthy" lifestyle for many years. It is definitely going to be a challenge to start making the choices that will get you back on the road to health and wellness. While every day passes, as long as we keep making better choices as far as diet, exercise, and attitude are concerned, we will slowly but surely be feeling better and getting more out of life. One quote that has always stuck with me is, "Living is hard, and dying is easy." In my years in private practice, I have treated many patients who were looking to get more out of life, and I have used this quote frequently in trying to get people to really start working at living.

If you sit back and think about it, dying really is easy. I don't want to mean "dying" in a literal sense but, to me, dying means that you have a horrible quality of life. Now, it is really easy to drive through the local fast-food burger place two to three times per day for meals, and stop at the soda machine for some empty calories at snack time throughout the day, but we all know where this will get us. On the other hand, it is much harder to plan on living and make those healthier decisions that we all know we should be making if we want to play with our grandchildren and great-grandchildren someday. This book will make it much easier for you to make those tough decisions on a day-to-day basis.

It is up to each one of us how we want to feel when we reach 65, 75, 95, or, dare I say, 110 years old. Researchers are now predicting that we should be living to 125 years old. As my good friend and colleague, Dr. Eric Plasker, stated in his bestseller, *The 100 Year Lifestyle,* "If you are a baby boomer, you'll join the nearly 400 million people around the world who will be 100 years of age or older by 2050 and the estimated 2 million centenarians in the United States alone." Maybe the most powerful statement in Dr. Plasker's book is: "The truth is your body has the hardware to live to 100 years and beyond."[1] Just take a minute and really think about this: what do we need to start doing today, so we can enjoy this century that we are about to live? Do we really want to rot like a vegetable the last twenty to thirty years of our life, or do we want to enjoy them?

Take a look at the excerpt on page nine and ten and decide which scenario you would rather have as you age. I have definitely seen both scenarios in my chiropractic practice. I know what I want when I reach that age; you have to decide what you want for your life. For me, the choice is easy, but it takes willpower, dedication, continued learning, and maybe help from your significant other, friends, family, coworkers, and heath/wellness care providers. We must remember that this isn't a fad diet, a month or two of hitting the gym, a New Year's resolution, or a short-term change for bikini season. This is a lifestyle that we can adopt to ensure the best possible life we can have.

Detoxify Your Lifestyle Quiz – Motivation Gauging Where You are Today

1. How long do I want to live?
A. 65-75
B. 76-85
C. 86-100
D. 101 +

2. How long would I want to live if I felt great?
A. 65-75
B. 76-85
C. 86-100
D. 101 +

3. I feel my current lifestyle will get me a great quality of life as I age.
A. no way
B. I need serious changes
C. it's OK most of the time
D. I have a great lifestyle

4. I would rate my health compared to friends/family who are roughly the same age as:
A. I am much unhealthier
B. they seem a little healthier
C. I'm a little healthier
D. I am much healthier than my peers

5. I eat out ____ times per week:
A. 10 or more times
B. 5-9 times
C. 1-4 times
D. almost never

6. I eat _____ servings of vegetables per day:
A. 0
B. 1-4
C. 5-7
D. 8 or more

7. I supplement with vitamins, fish oil, and other nutrients and minerals daily:
A. I take nothing
B. I take a multivitamin sometimes
C. I take a couple of vitamins most of the time
D. I take all essential nutrients on a daily basis

8. I would rate my home and work stress levels as:
A. I am always very stressed out
B. I have to work at it daily
C. I can control my stress fairly well
D. my life is very peaceful and stress free

9. I exercise:

A. only when I have to walk up my stairs
B. a couple of times a month
C. a couple of times a week.
D. 5-6 times per week – No exceptions

10. I eat breakfast:

A. never
B. 0-2 times per week
C. 3-5 times per week
D. 6-7 times/week

Now add up your score with A=1, B=2, C=3, D=4

0-17 – Time to really take a look at your life and make some drastic changes.

18-25 – I've definitely seen worse, but it's time to commit to making some changes.

26-33 – Seem to be doing things OK, if we just tweak some lifestyle changes you will be on your way to health and longevity.

34 or above – You seem to be in great health already; by reading this book, you can learn a few more things to really take your lifestyle to the next level of health and longevity.

Which Life Would You Choose at Eighty Years Old?

Scenario 1

*No aches or pains as you get out of bed every morning.
*An abundance of energy every day.
*Able to play with and enjoy your grandchildren.
*Walk with your significant other every morning.
*Continue to golf three times per week.
*Hike up the Rocky Mountains if your heart desires.
*Still enjoying great sex.
*No need for medications or surgeries.
*Never get sick.
*Feel motivated to learn and experience new opportunities.

Scenario 2

*Can barely get out of bed in the morning.
*Need two pots of coffee before you can
remember what day it is.
*Stuck on couch all day long because it hurts too
much to get off it.
*Have to remember to take a cocktail of
medications every morning and night.
*Have four doctor appointments every week, and
cannot understand why you feel like crap.
*With all of your doctors, you cannot understand
why you are chronically sick.
*No energy or motivation to do anything.
*Feel like your life isn't worth living anymore.

I wrote this book with one major premise in mind. It is a quote I tell my patients every day, "If it wasn't here five hundred years ago, then do not put it in your body today." I pose this question to myself every time I go the grocery store. Was this soda here five hundred years ago? How about this frozen pizza? Were fast-food cheeseburgers here when our ancestors were alive? If the answer is no, then we should definitely stay away from it. If we could simply live by this rule even 85-90 percent of the time, we could drastically reduce many of the old-age, degenerative diseases that plague America today. Each chapter in this book will always get back to what our ancestors did, whether that pertains to our foods, our exercises, or even our stress levels. I would advise you to write this quote down, put it on your fridge and read it every day. Next time you feel like grabbing a soda or other sugary snack, just ask yourself, "Were sodas around five hundred years ago?"

Each chapter is broken down into some of the key health and wellness tidbits that we can immediately integrate into our busy, hectic lifestyles. I am not saying that we have to do everything every single day, but adopting a few healthy habits will bring us years of good health and wellness. Another

point I want to make before we get started
is to not be discouraged when you fall off
the wagon. We all fall off the wagon. No
big deal, just get back in the saddle. Get
refocused, reenergized, and recommit
yourself to the lifestyle you want. It's going to
be hard in the beginning, but the first week
will turn into the first month, the first month will
turn into a few months, and a few months
will turn into your first full year of taking back
your health, wellness, and longevity. Because
we know that everyone falls off the wagon,
we should all start slowly, and we encourage
cheat days or, as I like to call them, "reward"
days.

So whatever your motivation may be, I
want to congratulate you again by taking
one of the many steps to your health and
longevity. It's a great ride, and I enjoy having
you along with me to get the most out of it. I
look forward to meeting you someday in the
near future and having you share your story
with me.

Start Detoxifying Your Lifestyle Now

Motivation

1. Commit to turning your lifestyle around today!
2. Write your goals down on paper about what lifestyle choices you are going to change!
3. Write down how you plan to implement those changes this week!
4. Share with friends and family your new lifestyle goals and invite them to join you!
5. Give yourself one reward or "cheat" day per week! You must earn it though.
6. Get your significant other or friends to commit to detoxifying their lifestyle with you!

Lifestyle Habit 2
Fats – Which ones are we supposed to eat?

Such a scary word: "fat." Are you shaking already? No need to worry; fat is an essential nutrient that we must eat. In fact, a lot of us are actually deficient in it. Did you know that your brain is actually made up of a fatty acid called docosahexaenoic acid (DHA)? Or you might have heard of it called omega-3 or fish oil. Almost all of us are deficient in this very essential and important nutrient. One big misconception that we all have is that eating fat makes us fat. This isn't necessarily true. As we will talk about in the next chapter, sugar is the main culprit causing the obesity epidemic in America. Fat just gets a lot of the blame because a lot of us do not know any better, and the blame has to be put somewhere. There are many different kinds of fats. Good fats, bad fats, big fats, small fats, healthy fats, and unhealthy fats. I'll start by showing you all the different kinds, where they come from, and what they do in your body. We will then spend a little time on the bad fats, and a little more time on the good fats. I don't like to dwell on the negative stuff in any aspect of life. I would much rather educate you about the good, essential fats out there that we need to get in our diets on a daily basis. I'll then show you that we, as humans, should be consuming all these different kinds of fats. Finally, we'll look at a few charts on foods that will give us a good shot at getting the most "good" fats in our diet.

Detoxify Your Lifestyle Quiz – Fats

1. How many meals per week do you eat fried foods?
A. 0

B. 1-3

C. 4-6

D. 7 or more

2. How many meals per week do you eat wild fish?
A. 7 or more

B. 4-6

C. 1-3

D. 0

3. How many meals per week do you cook with olive oil or coconut oil?
A. 7 or more

B. 4-6

C. 1-3

D. 0

4. Do you know the difference between good and bad fats?
A. yes

B. A little

C. no

5. Do you currently take a fish oil supplement?
A. all the time
B. sometimes
C. never

6. Do you regularly eat different types of nuts such as almonds, walnuts, pecans, etc.?
A. every day
B. occasionally
C. rarely
D. never

7. How often do you eat red meat per week?
A. 0
B. 1-3
C. 4-6
D. 7 or more

8. Do you buy grass-fed organic meats?
A. always
B. sometimes
C. rarely
D. never

Now add up your score with: A=3, B=2, C=1, D=0

*0-6 – You are eating too many of the wrong types of fats and not enough of the good fats. This can lead to many health problems right now or in the future. Continue to read and study this chapter to see what you can do to *detoxify your lifestyle*.

7-13 – You are getting some of the right types of fat in your diet, but you could definitely use some improvement with regard to good vs. bad fats. Study this chapter and become a much better shopper.

14-19 – You are doing fairly well with your diet. Just keep adding more and more good fats in your diet and you will continue to reap the benefits.

20-24 – You understand the different types of fats and are doing well with your diet. Continue to read about fats and enjoy the benefits of a healthy lifestyle.

Types of Fats

Type of Fat	Foods	Health Promoting or Health Risk
1. Trans Fat	Partially Hydrogenated oils	Increase risk of heart disease
	Fast food	Increase bad cholesterol
	Snack food	Decrease good cholesterol
	Fried food	
2. Saturated Fat	Meats	Increases bone health
	Dairy	Strengthens immune system
	Butter	Cell membrane health
	Coconut and palm oil	(consume in moderation)
	Some vegetables	

3. Unsaturated
   Fats

A. Omega -6s	Flaxseed	Skin and hair health
	Whole-grain breads	Regulates metabolism
	Nuts	
	Cereals	
B. Omega-3s	Fish	Cardiovascular health
	Organic meats	Brain health
	Nuts	Reduces Alzheimer's
		Reduces depression/ anxiety

Trans Fats

Let's start with the worst fat out there, trans fat. In my mind, trans fat is basically just a poison, and often labeled as its alias— "partially hydrogenated oils." Again, it wasn't here five hundred years ago, and it definitely shouldn't be here now or consumed by us. Basically, trans fats are produced when you hydrogenate oil for the purpose of making the oil more solidified. Manufacturers like this because it increases the shelf life of the fat. Trans fats are also commonly found in our fried foods such as the most common vegetable consumed by kids here in America—French fries. This stat makes no sense to me. How can French fries be the most common vegetable consumed by our children? We all know French fries are not good for us. As parents, why do we keep letting our children consume fries over and over? We need to stop this behavior immediately and show our children a better diet.

We cannot forget about fried chicken either. Other common places we'll find trans fats are in cookies, cakes, doughnuts, and other pastries. So what makes this fat so bad? Let's name a few of the effects trans fat has on our body. For starters, it increases LDL cholesterol, which is the bad cholesterol. It also lowers HDL cholesterol, which is our good cholesterol. So it does a double whammy as far as cholesterol is concerned. It may increase our risk for cardiovascular disease and stroke, and has also been shown to increase risk for type II diabetes. Do we really need any more reason to quit consuming trans fat? It has an enormous negative effect on America's biggest killer—cardiovascular disease. This isn't rocket science; let's just say NO to fried foods starting today and obviously cut down on our doughnuts and pastries as well. Not only because of the sugar content, but because we now know they contain this poison we know as trans fat.

Luckily for our future and us, America is waking up to the very serious health risks of trans fat. Many restaurant chains across America are eliminating all trans fats from their menus or at least drastically reducing them. Entire cities such as New York City have banned trans fats from their fast-food restaurants, and Chicago is considering doing the same. It is just a matter of time before the rest of the world wakes up and completely eliminates trans fats altogether. It is just great that the general public is demanding these changes for the betterment of the health of

America. All this can take place only when we, the people, demand it. Trust me—when large corporations make a change like this it is because of us. I commend you again for wanting a better life for yourself and taking the steps toward real health and wellness.

Saturated Fat

Next on the totem pole of fats is saturated fat. Saturated fat is the fat found in foods from animal meats and skin, dairy products, and some vegetables. This is going to be hard for a lot of us to "swallow," but based on Rule #1 (if it wasn't here 500 years ago, should you really be eating it today), would you suggest that saturated fats are OK to consume? Do you think our great ancestors ate animal meats and dairy products? Of course they did. They probably weren't eating the size steaks that we are accustomed to today, but they were definitely eating their portion of saturated fat from meat. It is absolutely OK to eat these foods in moderation. Unlike sugars and trans fats, I am not going to tell you to eliminate saturated fat. In fact I am going to encourage you to consume saturated fat in proper portion sizes. As long as our saturated fat comes from organic, healthy food sources that do not contain trans fats, I give it the OK to consume.

As a matter of fact, there are some documented benefits of saturated fat. A good portion of our cell membranes is made from this kind of fat. Cell membrane health is essential for our overall well-being. Saturated fat plays an important role in our bone health, as well as our immune system. It also serves as an antiviral and antifungal agent. By all means, do not be afraid of eating organic, red meat such as steak. Just do not eat the bread with the meal or other carbohydrates.

Unsaturated Fat

Let's now get into one of my favorite topics, unsaturated fats. These include monounsaturated and polyunsaturated fats. These are the good fats that we need to be getting in our diets every day. There are two main ones we need to spend a little bit of time getting to know and they are called omega-3s and omega-6s.

Dietary sources of omega-6s include cereals, nuts, whole grain breads, and almost all vegetable oils including corn oil and soy oil, baked goods, eggs, and poultry. As you can see, we get enough or most likely more than enough omega-6 fatty acids in our diet. Too much of this fat can become a problem. The omega-3 fats are from our fish, walnuts, almonds, flax, and organic, grass-fed animals. This is what we are severely deficient in. I will just come out and say it right now; we all need to be taking a fish oil capsule on a daily basis.

A good ratio of omega-6 to omega-3 is somewhere between 3:1 to 1:1. Our ancestors, centuries ago, had a diet with a ratio of 1:1. The westernization of our diets now has that ratio of around 20:1. Many studies have shown and many scientists believe that this high ratio is the cause for the high incidence of heart disease, obesity, inflammation, type II diabetes, and cancer. It also speeds up the aging process.

Have you been "fishing" for a solution to cardiovascular disease? Scientists first learned about the importance of omega-3s when they observed the Greenland Eskimos and their diets. Their diets consisted of a high-fat diet, mainly of fatty fish, but this population of Eskimos had a very low incidence of heart disease and arthritis. Now how could this be? We have been taught throughout the years that fat equals heart disease. Well, it's a little more complicated than that. First, what type of fat and, second, as we will learn in the next chapter, sugar is a big, big culprit as well. After observing the Eskimos, many studies soon came out showing the great benefits of omega-3 fats from fish. Let's go through a little of the research to see just how important fish oil capsules are, and then give you a little time to go out and buy your first bottle of fish oil capsules and start taking them tonight.

An article in *Archives of Internal Medicine* showed that taking omega-3s actually worked better than taking statin drugs as far as cardiac mortality is concerned.[2] Fish oil is something natural that has no known side effects, and works even better than one of the best-selling drugs in America. Take your choice of what you would rather have in your body.

There are a few mechanisms that omega-3s combat cardiovascular disease. First, they are anti-inflammatory, which is very important, as a lot of us are in a chronically inflamed state due to our westernized diets. They will improve the lining of our blood vessels, as well as fight blood clots. Omega-3s will also lower our blood pressure naturally and lower our triglyceride levels naturally.[3] Do we really need more reasons to rush out and get a bottle of high-quality fish oil capsules right now? With cardiovascular disease being one of the top killers in America, why take any chances? Start taking fish oil today and just make it part of your lifestyle. We all want to age gracefully, and without our heart and cardiovascular system, we just won't be able to do that.

With heart disease out of the way, let's talk about another major killer, cancer. Guess what, fish oil to the rescue. Fish oil suppresses cancer by several different mechanisms including decreasing oncogenes. Oncogenes are genes that code for a protein that is believed to cause cancer. Fish oil will help knock that out. As fish oil decreases inflammation levels throughout the body, it will also be drastically decreasing the chances of cancer. I think we all get the point—start taking fish oils today. Of course, this is one of the nutrients I think we do need to be supplementing with, but you can also get your omega-3s in your diet.

Wild salmon, mackerel, cod, herring, anchovies, and sardines are a few of the oily fish that contain a good amount of omega-3s. These fish have a much higher concentration of omega-3 to omega-6—probably around seven times as much, which is just great for our diet, which usually is more abundant in omega-6s. When buying fish, you must make sure your fish is wild and not farm raised. The farm-raised fish is fed grain, not the natural algae from the ocean that fish is supposed to feed on. When these fish are fed grain, they have a higher value of omega-6s. This takes away from the whole purpose of eating the fish. So make sure the package says "wild" and not "farm raised."

What can high-omega-3 foods do for you?

1. Reduce chronic inflammation throughout your body.

2. Keep your blood from clotting excessively.

3. Maintain the fluidity of your cell membranes.

4. Lower the amount of lipids (fats such as cholesterol and triglycerides) circulating in the bloodstream.

5. Decrease platelet aggregation, preventing excessive blood clotting.

6. Inhibit thickening of the arteries.

7. Increase the activity of endothelium-derived nitric oxide, which causes arteries to relax and open up.

8. Reduce atherosclerosis.

9. Reduce the risk of becoming obese and improve the body's ability to respond to insulin by stimulating the secretion of leptin, a hormone that helps regulate food intake, body weight, and metabolism.

10. Help prevent cancer cell growth.

Our poultry, beef, and other meats are also supposed to contain omega-3 fats in them. Just like fish, if animals ate the diet they are supposed to, they will in fact contain good amounts of essential omega-3 fats. Unfortunately, almost all the meat we buy at our traditional grocery stores comes from animals that were fed grain. These animals are supposed to graze on grass throughout their lifetime. Studies show grain fed animals decrease the amount of omega-3s while increasing total trans and saturated fat levels. Research also has suggested grass-fed cows have a natural ratio of omega-6 to Omega-3 at 1.8 to 1.0.[5] This is probably just what our ancestors' ratio was years ago, and our ancestors had hardly any incidences of heart disease. Does it now make sense to get grass-fed, organic meat and poultry? There are many companies online where you can get this type of meat, but the best way to get this, in my opinion, is to buy locally raised animals from local farmers. Another point about grass-fed, organic meats is these animals are not given antibiotics and steroids to fatten them up. Think about it, if the animals are give antibiotics and steroids and we eat the animals—what are we eating? We will be consuming the remnants of those toxic chemicals right inside our mouths. Once again, I bet our meat and poultry products weren't give antibiotics and steroids five hundred years ago, and five hundred years ago I bet our animals grazed on grass, and were not fed grain.

Some other sources of omega-3s are pecans, walnuts, almonds, and hazelnuts. These all make great snacks that we can munch on throughout the day. I really cannot think of a better little snack to have midmorning or afternoon when your stomach starts to rumble at the office. Instead of reaching for that sugary snack or soda, grab a handful of nuts or seeds and a nice cold glass of purified water or green tea. Instead of damaging our health with sugar, we are fulfilling our body's needs and our cravings with an essential nutrient such as omega-3 fat. All in all, we will feel more satisfied because the body is getting what it needs and we will even have more energy than if we'd consumed a caffeine-laden drink and some sugar. A soda and candy bar might spike our energy for about twenty minutes but we will soon crash. Putting in some omega-3s will actually fuel our bodies for a much longer time and get us over the hump for the rest of the day. As we continue to *detoxify our lifestyle*, we will soon notice that we don't even get drowsy spells midday at the office anymore. Some people will notice this in a couple of weeks, for others it will take a few months. It all depends on where your overall health is at the present time. Do not be discouraged if it takes longer than what you expected. Just keep making good choices; your time will come and your body, health, wellness, and quality of life will thank you later.

Specific Conditions Fish-Oil Supplementation Will Help with:

*Depression
*Cardiovascular disease
*Type II Diabetes
*Fatigue
*Dry, itchy skin
*Brittle hair and nails
*Inability to concentrate
*Joint pain
*High blood pressure
*Anxiety
*ADD/ADHD
*Alzheimer's disease
*Asthma
*Excessive menstrual pain
*High cholesterol
*Osteoporosis
*Compromised immune system
*Fatigue
*Epilepsy
*Cancer patients who cannot
maintain a healthy weight
*Rheumatoid arthritis
*Artherosclerosis
*Crohn's disease
*Ulcerative colitis
*Bipolar disorder

How to Get Essential Omega-3 Fats in Your Diet[4] (omega-3 concentration in grams)

Food Source	Serving Size	Grams of omega-3
Cod liver oil[1]	Tbsp	2.8
Walnuts	1 oz[2]	.6
Mackerel	4 oz	2.2
Flaxseeds	1 oz	1.8
Sardines	4 oz	1.8
Salmon	4 oz	1.7
Swordfish	4 oz	1.7
Scallops	4 oz	0.5
Soybeans	½ cup	0.5
Shrimp	4 oz	0.37
Pecans	1 oz	0.3
Broccoli	1 cup	0.2
Raspberries	1 cup	0.12
Spinach	½ cup	0.1
Kale	½ cup	0.1

Start Detoxifying Your Lifestyle Now

Fats

1. Eliminate all fried foods from your diet starting immediately!

2. Read labels more carefully, and do not buy or consume any trans fat or partially hydrogenated oil.

3. Start taking a fish oil capsule today!!

4. Eat fish at least two to three times per week. Make sure you buy wild fish instead of farm-raised fish.

5. Start buying more organic grass-fed meats, which will contain a healthier ratio of omega-3 fats.

6. When cooking with oil—start exclusively using extra virgin olive or coconut oil.

7. Snack on walnuts, pecans, almonds, and other nuts and seeds throughout the day.

Lifestyle Habit 3
Sugars

Cutting out unwanted sugars from our diet might be the absolute hardest thing we have to do. Sugar is probably the biggest addiction in America and the number one cause of many of our age-related degenerative diseases. Most of these "old-age" diseases can be 100 percent avoided if we could just keep our sugar in check. Much easier said than done. It is going to take a lot of willpower and dedication to keep our sugar intake at a tolerable level. Once we get used to cooking and eating without this nasty little substance, we will soon see the benefits in our quality of life and our health will drastically improve. Sit back and think about it—thousands of years ago all we ate were fruits, veggies, animal meats, as well as nuts and seeds. We did not have the abundance of breads, carbohydrates, processed foods, drinks, and sugars at our fingertips. Once again, if it wasn't here five hundred years ago, we are probably not supposed to eat it today. Trust me—sugar was not this readily available five hundred years ago. Check out the excerpt on the next page to take a look at just a few of the problems that sugar can cause.

Think twice the next time you want to put sugar into your bloodstream.

Sugar is a major cause of obesity and cardiovascular disease.

Sugar can increase your blood pressure.

Sugar may weaken your immune system.

Sugar has been linked to the development of cancer.

Increased sugar will eventually cause your body to be insulin resistant.

Sugar can cause loss of energy and fatigue.

Sugar will cause premature aging.

Sugar can interfere with the absorption of nutrients and protein.

Sugar can cause hormonal imbalances.

Sugar may contribute to depression and cognitive impairment.

Sugar is very addictive.

Sugar can elevate the symptoms of attention deficit/hyperactivity disorder.

Sugar may cause arthrosclerosis.

Sugar may damage your DNA structure.

There are many more ways that sugar damages the human body, so why on earth would you keep feeding yourself, your family, and your children this nasty little substance? Please do yourself a favor, and drastically start to decrease the amount of sugar you consume on a daily basis. It will do wonders for your body, your health, and your longevity.

Now, there are many diets out there that try to cut out our sugars and carbohydrates from our daily meals. Most notably, the Atkins Diet switched a lot of people from the traditional carbohydrate diet to a diet made up of proteins and fats. This worked wonders for some people, but after a while your sugar tooth comes back and you start to indulge yourself again.

The word "diet" never really caught on with me. That name alone suggests it is something you do for an allotted amount of time, see some results, and then go back to what you have been doing for the past couple of decades. I just don't like that word—diet. We really need to make a lifestyle change, and this can occur only if we are really committed to a health and wellness lifestyle.

Back to traditional diets that tell you to cut out all sugars at once. This always fails, because we need to slowly wean your sugar tooth down. Just like any addiction, if you cut something out too fast there will be consequences. When I first started in practice, I was caught in the dilemma that I wanted to help everyone right now, very quickly. I was urging my patients to go home and quit their current way of life today. We must realize as individuals, exactly how bad our diet is at this point in time, where our health is compared to where it realistically should be, and how quickly we want to change. This is different for everyone, and in private practice I have been very good at judging where people are at along their journey. If we need to start off slowly, then let's just eliminate one soda a day for the first month. If another individual has already cut out all breads, pastas, rice, and sweets, then obviously he or she is much more committed and willing to take the next step and we can push that individual along a little faster on the road to health. So we need to really sit down, gauge where we are, set some goals down in writing, and then get to work. Start by taking the survey on the next page to see where you rank on the sugar addiction scale.

Detoxify Your Lifestyle Exercise – Sugar/Carb Addiction Scale

1. How many slices of bread do I eat per day?
A. 0
B. 1-3
C. 4-6
D. 7 or more

2. How many servings of pasta per week?
A. 0
B. 1-3
C. 4-6
D. 7 or more

3. How many mornings per week do I eat cereal?
A. 0
B. 1-3
C. 4-6
D. 7 or more

4. How many sodas per day?
A. 0
B. 1-3
C. 4-6
D. 7 or more

5. How many other drinks besides water per day?

A. 0

B. 1-3

C. 4-6

D. 7 or more

6. For coffee drinkers: Do you drink black or add sugar and/or cream?

A. Black

C. Sugar or cream

7. How many salads do you eat per week?

A. 7 or more

B. 4-6

C. 1-3

D. 0

8. When feeling sluggish, I reach for:

A. fruits/veggies

B. protein bar

C. candy bar

D. soda fruit juice.

9. How many fast-food meals per week:

A. 0

B. 1-3

C. 4-6

D. 7 or more

10. How often do I read labels when grocery shopping.

A. 100 percent
B. Most of the time
C. Rarely
D. Never

Now add up your score with A=0, B=1, C=3, D=4

*0-9 – You sparingly consume sugars/carbs and are on your way to a very healthy lifestyle.

*10-19 – You are doing fairly well with your sugar/carb consumption. This book should educate you on how to simply tweak your diet and take your health, wellness, and longevity to the next level.

*20-29 – You definitely need some work and more education about sugars/carbs. Continue reading this book and start to make goals on how to reduce sugar/carb consumption.

*30-40 – Right now you are consuming way too many sugars/carbs, and it is most likely having a negative effect on your health and well-being. Start to make goals and put steps in place to slowly but surely start to reduce your sugar/carb consumption.

Let's get down to the nuts and bolts of what sugar really is. The only real function of sugar, or carbohydrate, is to provide the body with energy. Since proteins and fats already do that, there is really no need for dietary sugar, besides satisfying your sweet tooth and causing multiple diseases in the meantime. So where do we get our sugars from? Most people believe we get our sugars only from cakes, candies, and cookies. This is very far from the truth. Sugar, or glucose, is hidden all over our kitchen; most notably in our drinks (basically anything besides water), our breads, cereals, rice, sauces, dressings, condiments, and even in our fruit. Of course the sugar in fruit, fructose, is much healthier for you than other sugars, including glucose. Fruit sugar is very natural and easy on our bodies. Also, if you're eating whole fruit, you will also be digesting other minerals and nutrients that help with the digestion and elimination of that fructose sugar.

Humans have been eating fructose (in the form of fruit) for thousands of years. Fructose is readily absorbed and rapidly metabolized by the human liver. This is a very good thing because we do not want sugar in our bloodstream for very long. Also, in contrast to glucose, fructose does not stimulate insulin release in the body.[6] Unfortunately, westernized diets have resulted in significant increases in added fructose, leading to our obesity epidemic. This form of fructose is high-fructose corn syrup, or HFCS. There is nothing natural about HFCS. We will get to how nasty HFCS is in a little bit, but eating all natural sugars from fruit is perfectly fine. Another great example of how nature always knows what's best. Yes, our creator put sugar in our fruits, but he also put in just the right amount of nutrients to help absorb, use, and digest fructose. Don't mess with nature, and nature won't mess with us.

What happens when sugar, or glucose, enters our mouth and gets swallowed up? Well, when sugar enters our bloodstream, our pancreas immediately secretes insulin. In short, insulin's job is to take that sugar molecule and pull it into a cell so the body can use it. What happens when we bring in an overabundance of sugar at one meal or snack? The pancreas, as great as it is, just cannot keep up with our sugary foods and drinks. It may take up to hours before the pancreas can produce enough insulin to help rid our bloodstream of sugar. So in the meantime, sugar is just cruising around the bloodstream wreaking havoc. These free-floating sugars think it's fun to damage our tissues, blood vessels, and organs. Now imagine this occurring every single day for a few decades. This damage will finally build up and we will start feeling the consequences and degeneration (aging) that has happened to our body.

With the American diet, our little pancreas just cannot get a break, because before we know it, we have drank another soda or eaten another slice of bread. As much as our pancreas wants to fight for us, it finally gets burned out and cannot produce proper amounts of insulin anymore. When this happens, we are said to have insulin resistance. Before you know it, you have metabolic syndrome or type II diabetes. This is probably the biggest epidemic in America.

In my opinion, type II diabetes, or high blood sugar, might just be the cause of every degenerative condition that most Americans come across as they age. This is why I put so much emphasis on really cleaning out our kitchens of all the sugars, carbs, and grains. Type II diabetes has been linked to heart disease, strokes, cancers, common colds/flu, weakened immune system, depression, etc.

The *British Medical Journal*, in 2003, reported that insulin resistance is positively associated with diabetes and cardiovascular disease.[7]

I can state study after study and bore you to death of all the problems that can happen if we do not keep our carbohydrate intake at a low level. Why haven't we heard this information before? Well, I believe most physicians just do not grasp how bad sugars really are and how they, for lack of a better term, beat our bodies up.

This is why Dr. Joseph Mercola states on his very popular health and wellness Web site, www.mercola.com, that getting your insulin tested and stabilized is one of the first things you should do in order to get back on track to health. Dr. Mercola also states that the number one way to avoid premature aging is to avoid sugars and grains.[8] Insulin testing is one of the great diagnostic tests we can use to see how aged you really are. One study that backs up these last statements points out that, "Insulin reduction doubles longevity."[9] If we want to reduce insulin levels, we must reduce our sugar, carbohydrates, and grain intake. So I will go ahead and state that sugar/grain reduction can in fact double your longevity.

Probably the biggest culprit in our kitchens today is high-fructose corn syrup, or HCFS. Check your labels, people, it is everywhere. When you see this on the label—throw it away. So exactly what is HFCS? High-fructose corn syrup is basically corn syrup that has been processed to increase the sugar content and then mixed with glucose to reach its final form. What the heck sounds natural about that? A trend we have seen is that as our foods became more processed and increased HFCS, our sugar consumption actually decreased. So we are substituting one evil for a worse evil. America is actually flooded with high-fructose corn syrup. Time to start reading labels a little more closely, and really eliminate this stuff from our diet. HFCS has a huge influence on our obesity epidemic here in America.

In conclusion about sugars, let's really start to minimize and decrease our sugars starting today. Our first step should be measuring and gauging how much we are consuming. You will probably be very surprised, when you sit down and add up your entire day from breakfast toast or sugary cereal, to a morning snack, to your sandwich and soda at lunch, the afternoon pop and snack, your usual dinner with rolls, rice, etc., and, of course, an evening snack. Once we get a good grasp on how many carbohydrates we are actually eating, it is then time to determine the easiest way start eliminating them. Remember to go slowly. Maybe start with substituting bottled water for your afternoon soda, or a salad instead of the usual sandwich you have for lunch. Whatever you decide, just take baby steps and keep your overall goal in mind. Have faith, and if you have a setback, just know that tomorrow is a new day, and a new day brings new choices. It's up to you how long you want to live and more importantly the quality of life you want to have as you age.

Start Detoxifying Your Lifestyle Now

Sugars

1. Count your sugar and carbohydrate intake for one week in order to realize how much sugar you're actually consuming.

2. Eliminate soda, energy drinks, and other sugary drinks.

3. Drink your coffee black—no added sugar or cream.

4. Use lettuce wraps instead of bread when having a sandwich.

5. Eat whole fruit instead of sugary cereals, toast, and bagels for breakfast.

6. Eliminate sugary snacks such as cookies, candies, and other sweets.

Lifestyle Habit 4
Your Gut, Digestive Tract, and the Bacteria that Call it Home.

Intestinal flora, or gut bacteria, is the bacteria that line our intestinal tract. These are good bacteria that perform many of our body's functions. Healthy microorganisms that reside in the intestines, such as the lactobacilli species, form part of the body's defense system against food-borne pathogens and microorganisms. Without them, we could not survive. Don't get me wrong, there are definitely a lot of bad bacteria that we encounter every day through breathing, touching, and eating, but there are also millions of good bacteria that are inside our digestive tract. We actually have around ten times the amount of bacteria in our gut than we have cells in our entire body. These good bacteria inside of us are big players in our immune system. In order for us to have optimally functioning immune systems, we must have the right amount of good bacteria lining our digestive tracts. With the proper amount of good bacteria, we will have a much better chance of fighting off sickness and disease.

There are a number of lifestyle choices we make, such as our foods, medicines, drugs, alcohol, sugar, and other environmental toxins that wipe out the good bacteria in our intestinal tracts. When this happens, our body cannot function up to par and many symptoms and diseases can take over. In order to *detoxify our lifestyle*, we need to continually replenish our good bacteria so that our digestion can work properly. We can keep this community of bacteria thriving with a good diet, good health habits, and by supplementing with probiotics. Let's talk a little bit about how these very tiny, very busy organisms inhabit our digestive system and what can be done to help them flourish and in turn help keep us flourishing as we age gracefully.

In order for us to reach our maximum health and wellness, the tiny bacteria inside of us must be at their maximum health and wellness. How can the good bacteria get to this state? Good question—well, we need to first quit putting the killer toxins in our bodies, and replenish them with a probiotic supplement on a continual basis.

Some of the toxins that kill the bacteria are vaccinations and antibiotics. How many of these do our children go through just within the first few years of life? I have treated children in my practice who have had more rounds of antibiotics than I can count on both of my hands. What is the purpose of antibiotics—to kill bacteria, specifically bad bacteria that have caused some type of sickness or disease? I hate to break the news, but antibiotics don't have little radars on them that just go after the bad bacteria. They also wipe out the good bacteria in our digestive tracts. This is the reason why many young, sickly children stay that way. While children are trying to get over a sickness with antibiotics, they are also killing their good bacteria and therefore reducing the power of their immune systems. So before you know it, they are sick again, and given another round of antibiotics—are you starting to see the vicious cycle? I have a crazy idea—instead of giving our bodies something that is killing our good bacteria, and therefore making us weaker and more susceptible to sickness, why don't we take something that enhances our good bacteria, thereby enhancing our immune systems and overcoming the vicious cycle? This is when true health and wellness can occur, and we will not have to worry about getting sick again. Our children will be able to grow and develop properly without the use of drugs or surgeries. Just the way we were meant to.

Detoxify Your Lifestyle Quiz – Bacteria and your Digestive Tract

1. Are all bacteria bad?
A. yes
B. most all bacteria are bad.
C. a lot of bacteria are good for us.

2. Were you vaccinated as a child?
A. yes
B. not sure
C. no

3. How many rounds of antibiotics do you go through each year?
A. 5 or more
B. 3-4
C. 1-2
D. I absolutely stay away from antibiotics.

4. How often do you eat yogurt?
A. never
B. rarely
C. occasionaly
D. every day

5. How often do you get sick?
A. a lot
B. occasionally

C. rarely

D. never

6. How often do you suffer from diarrhea or constipation?

A. a lot

B. occasionally

C. rarely

D. never

7. Do you have at least two bowel movements per day?

A. never

B. rarely

C. sometimes

D. always

8. How often do you supplement with probiotics?

A. never

B. I have once or twice.

C. occasionally

D. I take probiotics regularly.

9. Have you ever done a colon flush?

A no way.

B. I'm thinking about it.

C. I have once or twice.

D. every six months to a year.

10. According to Chapter 3, are you addicted to sugar?

A. very much so.

B. I have a fair amount of sugar in my diet.

C. I eat sugar occasionally.

D. I hardly have any sugar.

Now add up your score with A=1, B=2, C=3, D=4

*__10-17__ – Your digestive system might not be working up to par. A healthy digestive tract is one of the keys to *Detoxifying Your Lifestyle*. Read on to find out how to improve your digestive tract.

__18-24__ – Your digestive tract needs a little work. Start eating some healthy foods that will restore your digestive tract.

__25-32__ – You already implement a lot of healthy lifestyle choices. Continue to read this chapter and take your digestive tract to the next level of health.

__33-38__ – Congratulations on a healthy digestive tract. Keep reading and stay motivated on your health and wellness journey!

To add to the problem of having our intestinal bacteria disrupted, sugar actually feeds the bad bacteria. So as we our living an unhealthy lifestyle that is killing our good bacteria, we keep eating our sugar diets and making the bad bacteria much stronger. Many health experts believe this is why we have sugar and carbohydrate cravings. All the unfriendly bacteria in our gut are craving sugar. Again, this can very quickly turn into a vicious cycle of cravings and binges. As you can see already, it is pretty difficult to keep our intestinal flora maintained. From wiping out the good bacteria to feeding the bad bacteria—we can quickly disrupt everything going on inside our intestines. Thankfully, it is not very hard to turn the switch on this problem and get our intestines working for us.

Besides helping our immune system, our good bacteria help us digest our food, absorb the nutrients from our gut, and help prevent allergies. The key component here is absorbing the good nutrients that we will be eating after reading this book. What is the point of eating good foods if our body cannot digest and absorb them? These good bacteria do just that. One of the first things we all need to do when *detoxifying our lifestyle* is making sure our gut bacteria are intact and working for us. Once our good bacteria are working for us, they will help get rid of the bad bacteria as well as reduce stomach irritation and inflammation.

What Our Friendly Bugs Do for Us!!

1. Greatly enhance our **immune system** and help protect us from sickness.
2. Regulate intestinal pH.
3. Protect us from pesticides and environmental pollutants.
4. Help prevent infection.
5. Cleanse the intestinal tract and colon, and help regulate bowel movements.
6. Help in our digestion process.
7. Help maintain healthy cholesterol and triglyceride levels.
8. Help prevent allergies.
9. Help clear up eczema.
10. Heal intestines from a variety of ailments.

Disruption of our intestinal flora has been linked with many conditions and diseases. In many studies, depression and anxiety have been linked to a disrupted digestive tract. Poor intestinal flora contributes to depression and anxiety symptoms by altering the immune system response. A lot of scientists and researchers actually call the gut the second brain. This is because most of the neurotransmitter serotonin is produced in your gut. Serotonin works specifically on our central nervous system to inhibit anger, anxiety, depression, and mood swings. As you can see, serotonin plays an important role in our emotional well-being. With over 90 percent of our serotonin being produced in our gut, it is very important that our gut is functioning properly. If our gut is not working up to par, we are much more prone to anger, depression, and anxiety issues. This might be hard to understand, but more and more research is now showing the link between anxiety-depressive disorders and digestive tract disturbances. In my clinic alone, I have noticed children and adults feeling much better emotionally when their diet is switched around. By supplementing with probiotics, depression and anxiety problems can be greatly diminished. Over the past few years, many health and wellness providers are now teaching patients how to change their diets and lifestyles to help with emotional diseases before turning to more invasive therapies.

As I mentioned earlier, one of the first things we need to do to *detoxify our lifestyle* is to reestablish our intestinal flora so our gut, intestines, and colon can do their jobs properly. We can accomplish this by taking a bottle of high-quality probiotics. Probiotics are a supplement of good, healthy bacteria. Pick up a bottle of probiotics from your health food market or wellness-care provider today. They usually need to stay refrigerated because they contain millions of live cultures of bacteria that will die if heated. These are the same live cultures of bacteria found in yogurt. Some health care providers believe you should be on probiotics on a daily basis for the rest of your life. This probably isn't a bad idea, but we can also get these "good" bacteria in our diets. Either way, we need to definitely keep replenishing our systems with good bacteria for the rest of our lives.

So how can we get good bacteria in our diet? Very easy and a great daily snack! Yogurt! High-quality organic yogurt tastes great and is great for us. I should also mention very essential for us to consume on a consistent basis. Look for yogurts in the natural foods section of your grocery store. Make sure they contain no artificial sweeteners and are low in sugars. My preference is for an assortment of fruits like blueberries, raspberries, and strawberries. Yogurt is very simple and easy to consume on a daily basis as part of our breakfast or midday snack. Another food high in good bacteria is sauerkraut. Sauerkraut is basically a fresh vegetable changed into one of the richest sources of good bacteria (lactobacilli) by the process of fermentation. These raw-cultured vegetables are key to restoring order to the digestive tract. Sauerkraut is also effective in treating peptic ulcers, ulcerative colitis, colic, food allergies, vaginal infections, constipation, and digestive disorders. I believe it does all this by simply returning the intestinal flora to a healthy state.

Other foods that we can include in our diet for intestinal health include cheeses, miso, tempeh, and kefir. I know the latter three are fairly rare and not normal in the standard American diet, but cheese, yogurt, and sauerkraut are fairly easy to consume on a regular basis. Remember to always eat all natural, organic foods whenever possible.

Probiotic Supplementation

When supplementing with a round of probiotics we usually don't feel anything different going on inside our body (unless you're fighting off diarrhea). Here is a list of functions that detoxifying with probiotics will perform and how it will help benefit us:

1. Probiotics will help boost immune response by inhibiting growth of pathogenic organisms.
2. Probiotics detoxify the intestinal tract by protecting intestinal mucosa levels.
3. Probiotics develop a barrier to food-borne allergies.
4. Probiotics neutralize antibiotic-resistant strains of bacteria.
5. Probiotics reduce cancer risk.
6. Probiotics reduce the risk of inflammatory bowel disease (IBS) and diverticulosis.
7. Probiotics synthesize needed vitamins for healing.
8. Probiotics prevent diarrhea by improving digestion.

Start Detoxifying Your Lifestyle Now

1. Stop feeding sugar to the bad bacteria in your gut.

2. Start detoxifying with probiotics. You can pick up a high-quality probiotic supplement from your local health food store or your wellness provider. This is one of the very best things you can do for your health, wellness, and longevity.

3. Make yogurt and sauerkraut part of your diet today!!

4. Consider getting a colon flush to help clean out your intestinal tract.

5. Avoid toxins and foods that wipe out your good intestinal flora.

Lifestyle Habit 5
Raw Foods and Greens

I would like to start this chapter out by talking a little bit about what our great, great ancestors used to eat years ago and what we are still supposed to eat today. I'll give you a hint—take a look at the title of this chapter. We all need to get back to the era of hunters and gatherers. The hunter-gatherer lifestyle basically consists of eating raw foliage, plants, vegetables, fruits, nuts, and seeds, and catching your own wild game to eat. This sounds like the perfect diet to me. It is basically what we should still be eating now. We can simply substitute buying our food at an organic health market for picking the food ourselves from the earth. Of course, there is nothing wrong with organic gardening in our backyard if that is what you like to do. I also want to mention that these hunter-gatherers were also on their feet all day walking, not sitting on a couch in front of a TV. So what have we learned from this previous lifestyle of our ancestors? They had a much lower risk of cardiovascular disease, diabetes, cancer, and obesity. They led a relatively simple life with little or none of the age-degenerative diseases that plague us today. They did not mess with nature. They ate and survived off the earth, just as it was intended to be.

Detoxify Your Lifestyle Quiz – Raw Foods and Greens

1. How many servings of fruit do you eat per day?
A. 8 or more
B. 5-7
C. 2-4
D. 1 or less.

2. How many servings of vegetables do you eat per day?
A. 8 or more
B. 5-7
C. 2-4
D. 1 or less.

3. Do you usually have a salad with your meal?
A. always
B. occasionally
C. rarely
D. never

4. How do you eat the majority of your vegetables?
A. raw
B. steamed
C. cooked

5. Do you have a garden that you eat out of?
A. yes
B. occasionally
C. rarely
D. no

6. Do you buy most of your groceries organic?
A. always
B. occasionally
C. rarely
D. never

7. Do you eat a rainbow of colors with regard to fruits and vegetables?
A. always
B. occasionally
C. rarely
D. never

8. Do you understand what genetically modified foods are?
A. yes
B. I think so.
C. not really.
D. never heard of genetically modified foods.

9. Do you consume red wine?
A. one glass per night.
B. a couple of times per week.

C. only on special occasions.

D. never

10. How many times per week do you eat out?

A. never

B. rarely

C. occasionally

D. always

Now add up your score with A=4, B=3, C=2, D=1

10-16 – Your diet is not getting the nutrients, vitamins, and minerals that you need for a long, healthy lifestyle. Read and study this chapter, and start implementing new foods into your lifestyle.

17-24 – You definitely need to be getting more fruits and vegetables into your diet. Read on to find out why these foods are so important.

25-32 – Your get a fair amount of the right foods in your diet. With a few simple changes in your daily intake, you will be on your way to a very healthy diet.

33-39 – Congratulations on consuming the right types of foods. Keep up the good work, and you will enjoy a long life of health and wellness!

In a perfect world, I would love to walk into my backyard and pick some raspberries, blueberries, and strawberries for breakfast. Along with that, I would pick a few oranges and squeeze a fresh glass of orange juice. For lunch and dinner, I would again pick some lettuce or spinach leaves from my backyard garden along with red peppers, carrots, and celery. Probably easier said than done, but that is exactly what our ancestors did for years. Of course they would also catch and eat wild game and fish as well. They would also often eat their meat uncooked. Eating raw meat now gets a bad rap because of the potential side effects it might have, but remember wild game eats off the land as well, and does not have unwanted bacteria, viruses, etc. Only when our agriculture system raises animals on a grain-fed diet with steroids and drugs do our animals become sick. Farmers believe we must fatten up our animal supply as quickly as possible in order to sell them at top dollar. We then eat all the drugs and steroids they are pumping into our animals. Probably not the healthiest choice.

With the development of agriculture came a decrease in the number of hunters and gatherers. This is also when a lot of our problems came into play. Agriculture and farming can be a very good thing if done properly, but in this day and age it's about the bottom dollar and not the health of our food supply. I already mentioned how we raise our animals, but our vegetation is just as bad. They are now spraying our crops numerous times throughout the season with chemicals that will eventually be consumed by us. Over one billion tons of pesticide products are used each year in the United States alone.

12 Foods with Most Pesticides

1. Peaches
2. Apples
3. Sweet bell peppers
4. Celery
5. Nectarines
6. Strawberries
7. Cherries
8. Pears
9. Imported Grapes
10. Spinach
11. Lettuce
12. Potatoes

12 Foods with Least Pesticides[10]

1. Onions
2. Avocados
3. Sweet corn
4. Pineapples
5. Mango
6. Asparagus
7. Sweet Peas
8. Kiwi
9. Bananas
10. Cabbage
11. Broccoli
12. Papaya

With all the pesticides and other chemicals sprayed on our crops, make sure you are consuming organic food as much as possible to limit your exposure to these toxic chemicals.

Producers have also genetically modified (GMO) many of our foods.

Many people do not understand what genetically modified foods are. The DNA in GMO foods has actually been altered. The purpose of altering the DNA in the seeds of various plants is to make the plant more resistant to pests and harsh environmental conditions.[11] Simply put, the DNA of seeds of GMO food is injected with pesticides, herbicides, fungicides, etc. in hopes that farmers can reduce spraying the crops with pesticides, herbicides, and fungicides. If the crops were sprayed, we would be able to rinse and wash off the pesticides, but with genetic modification we cannot wash off the toxic material because it is implanted into the DNA of the seed. This point brings us back to rule number one. Were genetically modified foods around five hundred years ago? Absolutely not! When cleaning out your kitchen (Chapter 6), please make sure you throw out all GMO foods. Of course, all natural, organic foods will not be genetically modified. So if we buy all organic produce, we will have nothing to worry about as far as genetic modification. Be very careful when shopping at your traditional grocery stores; some stats show that seven out of ten foods at the grocery store may be genetically modified or have an ingredient that is genetically modified. Some of the most common foods that are genetically modified are soy beans, corn, and tomatoes.

Most Common GMO Food. Be sure to read labels and buy Non-GMO Foods.

Soybeans
Corn
Tomatoes
Beets
Potatoes
Some oils
Wheat
Dressings
Condiments
Rice

Make sure you check the labels carefully for GMO ingredients in these foods:[12]

Infant formula
Bread
Hamburgers and hot dogs
Mayonnaise
Cookies
Candy
Chips
Meat substitutesIce
Frozen yogurt
Soy sauce
Tomato sauce
Baking powder
Confectioner's glaze
Vanilla
Peanut butter
Vanilla extract
Malt

Salad dressing
Cereal
Margarine
Crackers
Chocolate
Fried food
Veggie burgers
cream
Tofu
Soy cheese
Protein powder
Powdered sugar
Alcohol
Powdered sugar
Enriched flour
Pasta
White vinegar

Why is GMO food not the best choice? We cannot even fully understand the long-term effects of GMO foods because they have not been around that long, but we do have some information on possible side effects.

Some of the health problems already documented to be possibly caused by GMO foods include memory loss, hair loss, muscle weakness, muscle pain, and muscle spasm. GMO foods may also be carcinogenic, allergenic, and just plain toxic to our systems. Do we really want to risk our health, wellness, and longevity by consuming foods that have been genetically modified? I believe in the years to come, the results will finally show how dangerous the process of genetic modification will be—so much so, that Europe has already banned GMO foods. Since 1998, the European Union governments have not authorized GMO products. Of course, America is behind the times, and the only explanation I can come up with is the bottom dollar. Our food giants have the control until we, the people, speak out for our health and force the food giants to quit producing GMO foods. Start buying local, all natural, organic produce and foods and that is what the grocery stores will have to stock. It is up to us how healthy we want to be, how healthy we

RAW FOODS AND GREENS   85

want our children to be, and how healthy we want our country to be.

We need to be eating the rainbow every day. What I mean by this is we should be eating an assortment of fruits and vegetables every day. Make sure to hit every color of the rainbow. All fruits and vegetables contain essential vitamins and minerals. They also contain a new type of nutrient that many of us may not have heard of called "phytonutrients." Phytonutrients, or phytochemicals, as they are also referred to, are the active health-protecting compounds that are found in plants. "Phyto" means plant and, of course, we know what nutrient means. In my office, we refer to phytonutrients as plant nutrients. I continually tell my patients that we all need to be getting an abundance of plant nutrients on a daily basis. If we are not eating enough vegetables throughout the day, then there are plant nutrient supplements or drinks that we can be supplementing with. However, I always encourage people to try to get everything their bodies need in their diets as a first priority and then supplement as a last effort or insurance plan. I guess we could also refer to them as vegetable nutrients. Each color of plant or vegetable contains a different phytonutrient makeup, and all the colors are very beneficial. This is why we need to be eating an assortment of plants, vegetables, and fruits.

We have known for years that those people who eat a lot of fruits and vegetables are traditionally healthier and live a longer, healthier life. We always used to attribute this fact to fruits and vegetables having a lot of vitamins and minerals in them, but we now know that even more important than vitamins and minerals are the many phytonutrients they contain. Relatively speaking, this is actually a recent discovery. Every year we are discovering more and more phytonutrients in our fruits and vegetables.

When I think of phytonutrients and all the health-promoting benefits of them, I traditionally think of green food. With more and more research coming out about the anticancer and antiheart disease benefits of phytochemicals, I cannot stress enough how important vegetables are. Maybe Mom was onto something when she wouldn't let us leave the dinner table until we ate all our vegetables.

Phytonutrients are basically antioxidant, anti-inflammatory, and immune-boosting chemicals that are very powerful and promote many different functions in our bodies and in our cells. Hippocrates (460-ca. 377 BC), the father of medicine, was a Greek physician who used the leaves and bark of the willow tree to treat fevers. Even in that day and age, they knew how important and how powerful the phytonutrients from plants and greens were. Usually when you hear the word "superfood," it is classified as such because of its phytonutrient makeup. There are actually entire books dedicated to superfoods, and a good diet and lifestyle should be based around these types of foods. Phytonutrients help shield us from environmental toxins and repair damaged cells. From living your current lifestyle, do you think you can benefit from phytonutrients? I definitely think so. In my office, every patient is recommended two supplements no matter what. They are plant nutrients and a fish oil capsule. I believe everyone walking this earth can benefit from these two supplements. According to a study in the prestigious *Journal of American Medical Association (JAMA)*, "Current research shows that, at every step along the road to malignancy, plant chemicals tend to reduce the likelihood of transmission to the next stage."[13]

Our cells are bombarded with different stresses every day. Whether that stress is physical, emotional, or chemical, each cell in our body has to combat these stresses and try to survive. During the process of our cells combating these daily stresses, they form free radicals. We've all heard of free radicals before and know they are bad. They are basically the by-products of our cells' daily activities. If we have too many free radicals in our system, they can interact with our DNA or cell membranes and cause damage. Ingesting enough antioxidants can counteract or eat up these free radicals before they cause damage. We now understand how our fruit and vegetable phytonutrients act as antioxidants and help fight free radicals in our systems. There is no way we can stop the production of free radicals happening every day. Of course, we can decrease our stress levels and decrease the toxins in our bodies, but there will always be free radicals produced in our bodies on a daily basis. The more fruits and vegetables in our diets, the better our bodies can counteract free radicals and decrease the aging process. Taking a plant nutrient supplement will give us the added insurance that we are getting enough phytonutrients on a daily basis. One thing I must remind you though—taking a plant nutrient supplement is not a substitute for eating your vegetables, fruits, salads, etc. Just think of it as a little insurance.

Some different types of phytonutrients that you may have heard of before are isoflavone, lycopene, carotene, anthocyanin, lutein, and zeaxanthin. Remember, there are hundreds, if not thousands, of phytonutrients and I believe we have just discovered the tip of the iceberg with phytonutrients.

Another phytonutrient you probably have heard of is resveratrol. Resveratrol is a phytonutrient found in grapes and red wine. It is also found in different types of berries, but most prominently in grapes. It is actually most abundant in the grape skins. So make sure you are eating the entire grape and not just the inside. I am not an advocate of alcohol, although there have been many studies showing that one drink per day can actually be beneficial to our health and longevity. Actually, I have taken care of many elderly in my practice, and I always ask them what their secret is to their longevity. Almost always, I get two answers. One, all my elderly patients swear by drinking one glass of wine per night. Some of these patients admit to doing this for fifty to sixty years. With all the research out there now, we can show how powerful the phytonutrient resveratrol is, and some of these older patients of mine have been getting resveratrol in their diets for many years on a daily basis. The other answer my elderly patients always give me as their key to longevity is a positive attitude, and it definitely shows in these people.

You just cannot beat a positive outlook on life. These people just decide to be happy every day when they wake up. The choice really is ours, and we have the ability to make that choice every morning when we wake up. It might take some training and focus to do this, but just start your day off with a positive quote or affirmation. If that doesn't work, start the morning off with listing a few things you are thankful for. For me, this starts off in the shower every morning. I just relax and make the choice to be positive and in a great mood. As we all know, going to the workplace or getting the kids ready to go, whatever our daily activities may be, we are all going to be bombarded with stresses throughout the day. So let's at least start each and every day off on a good foot and make each day the best possible day imaginable. I've seen it work for so many of my patients while in private practice, and the older patients I meet are living testaments that a positive outlook on life and a happy-go-lucky demeanor will get you far in regard to health, happiness, and longevity.

I believe we will continue to discover more and more phytonutrients in our fruits and vegetables. As for now, just start eating as many fruits and vegetables as possible. Start eating from our earth. These foods grow here for a reason, and that reason is for us to consume. Our foods are not supposed to be made in a factory. Check out the list of superfoods that contain an abundance of phytonutrients. I urge you to get at least a couple of superfoods in each meal of the day. As for midmorning snacks and midafternoon snacks, why not make them superfoods as well?

Superfoods – Foods High in Phytonutrients

*Green Tea
*Blueberries
*Blackberries
*Strawberries
*Broccoli
*Cauliflower
*Spinach and other dark green leafy vegetables
*Purple grapes
*Kiwi
*Grapefruit
*Brussels sprouts
*Tomatoes
*Red and green peppers
*Pumpkin
*Carrot

When I first meet people they always tell me how they just don't have the time to cook healthy meals for themselves and their families. I usually respond with, you don't have enough time not to. It is just something we have to do if we want to *detoxify our lifestyle*, live healthy, and have a long fulfilling life without sickness and disease. The second thing I will say is that it takes no time at all to eat raw fruits and vegetables. No cook time, just put a tray on the kitchen counter and let everyone eat up. We should be eating the bulk of our food raw anyway. Since this is the case, I really just eliminated the excuse that "there is not enough time in the day to prepare healthy meals." How did our ancestors eat five hundred years ago? You guessed it—they ate, or should I say grazed on, raw foods all day long. This is just the way nature intended these foods to be eaten. They didn't have microwaves back then. I am not saying to throw out your microwaves and conventional ovens, but I am saying to slowly make raw foods a larger portion of your meals.

Why should we start to eat raw more than cooked foods? Well, cooking depletes a lot of the nutrients and minerals in the food. Enzymes in foods are specific types of proteins that help the digestion process and other metabolic activities that are very important inside the body. Cooking or processing our food depletes the essential enzymes in food, and the important biological functions of the enzymes cannot take place once we consume the food. Enzymes also enable the body to utilize vitamins and minerals. Simply put, heating foods will decrease the digestion process and make the food more toxic. Another benefit of raw foods is that the bacteria in certain types of foods that we talked about in Chapter 4 will be readily available. The good bacteria are very heat sensitive and will be killed with any heating or processing. Vitamins, nutrients, and phytonutrients are also injured because of the heat and left in an altered molecular state.

Overall, raw foods nourish and vitalize the body's inner environment. Eat the foods the way they were meant to be eaten. Once again, don't mess with nature and nature won't mess with us. Once you learn how to prepare healthy, raw meals that taste out of this world, you will never go back to some of your old cooking methods. I am not saying I eat a 100 percent raw diet, but I do incorporate a lot of raw foods in my meals. I love to grill just as much as the next guy, but that doesn't mean I cannot include a very healthy and bulky organic salad with my organic steak. Once you get used to it, it is very easy to incorporate raw foods on a daily basis, just as nature intended.

Start Detoxifying Your Lifestyle Now

1. Start eating a rainbow of fruits and vegetables every single day!

2. Eat a big percentage of your food raw!

3. Read labels very carefully for GMO foods and eliminate them.

4. Buy more food from your organic market or local farmer's market!

5. Incorporate superfoods into each meal!

6. Consume superfoods as your midday and midafternoon snacks.

7. One glass of red wine per night might be beneficial to you!

8. Prepare healthy meals at home as opposed to eating out.

9. Plan and write out a weekly meal plan in order to be prepared during your busy schedule. This will help eliminate consuming convenience foods throughout the week.

Lifestyle Habit 6
Cleaning out Your Kitchen

The first battle we have is to clean out our kitchens. I am not sure you can fathom how many toxins and junk foods are in your pantry and refrigerator right now. Don't get me wrong—it is much healthier to eat at home instead of going out to eat—but let's clean up our own kitchens before we can truly say "eating in is much healthier than eating out." We already talked about sugars and fats in previous chapters, but almost everything that comes in a box, can, or package is just loaded with sugars, artificial flavors, preservatives, and other junk and toxins. Do you really believe your body was meant to eat all this junk? Did our ancestors eat this stuff years ago? Back to the major premise of the book, "If it wasn't here five hundred years ago, we are probably not meant to eat it today." It is just a rule of thumb we should always live by, and if we do, we will be avoiding much of the junk that is in our diet and in our world right now. What do you think happens to your body after years of bombarding it with these processed sugars, flavors, preservatives, etc.? One of the main jobs of our liver, kidneys, and digestive tract is to eliminate unnecessary toxins. Now our cells, tissues, and organs are very good at detoxifying us, but that doesn't mean it is OK to keep dumping these toxins into our mouths. As an analogy, I regularly tell my patients, "Would you put dirty gasoline into your car?" I get a lot of weird looks and gestures and the answer is always no. The follow-up question is, of course, "Then why would you ever think about putting 'dirty' food or preservatives into your body's gas tank?"

Unfortunately, a lot of us take more pride in our automobile than we do our own health and wellness. It always amazes me that we take such great care of our cars and want longevity for our cars but couldn't care less about our own bodies. Let's face it, without our health and well-being, we are nothing. We all must realize that our health is our number one asset. So do not wait until a crisis to start to take care of your body and maintain it. Let's get our oil changed regularly, and always put high-quality octane into our tanks.

Now back to our kitchens. One of the first things we need to realize is how to quit eating all this processed junk. I know it makes it easier, especially when we are cooking for families, but simply start eating more fresh foods than boxed, canned, or processed foods. Go ahead and go through your kitchen right now and begin to throw away all the cans, boxes, and processed foods. After you notice there isn't much left in your kitchen, you can run off to your local health market or grocery store and pick up all the fresh fruit, vegetables, and organic meats and poultry that you desire. It is not hard at all to boil some veggies, cut up some fruit, or throw some all-natural, grass-fed poultry, beef, or pork on the grill. We can also use an assortment of herbs and spices for flavoring meats and other dishes. Natural herbs and spices have many health benefits as well.

This is not rocket science; just take a look at all the ingredients on a boxed or canned food item. Read through all the preservatives and unnatural junk that they put in this stuff. Did our ancestors eat all these chemicals? No wonder cancers, heart disease, and other longevity diseases plague America. We keep feeding these diseases with all the toxins and junk we put into our mouth. Let's just get back to eating fresh, natural foods. This one simple change will make a drastic improvement in your health. Check out the next page to take a look at just some of the health benefits of our common herbs and spices.

Rack up Health Benefits with these Herbs and Spices

Herb or Spice	Potential Health Benefit	Suggested Use
Basil	Antioxidant Decreases Inflammation	Tomatoes/Pesto Salads Marinades/ Sauces
Black Pepper	Stimulates Digestive System Stimulates Respiratory System	Meats Soups Salads, etc.
Chili	Antioxidant Increases Metabolism	Meat/Seafood Stews Dipping Sauces
Cilantro	Antioxidant Helps Digestion Natural Chelator	Latin/Mexican Cuisine Dipping Sauces Marinades/Rubs
Cinnamon	Lowers Blood Pressure Lowers Triglycerides	Good Substitute for Sugar Oatmeal

Dill	Antioxidant	Seafood
	Antimicrobial	Dipping Sauces
Garlic	Lowers Cholesterol	Marinades
	Antioxidant	Dressings
	Lowers Blood Pressure	Meats/Seafood Salads
	Boosts immunity	
Ginger	Antioxidant	Asian Cuisine
	Antimicrobial	Stir-fry
	Helps Osteoarthritis	Meats/Poultry/ Seafood
Lemongrass	Antioxidant	Seafood, Especially
	Anti-inflammatory	Shrimp Stir-fry
	Anticancer	Soups
Mustard Seed	Helps Stomachaches	Salads/Soups
	Helps Constipation	Meat/Poultry Dishes
Oregano	Antioxidant	Mediterranean Cuisine Salads
	Antimicrobial	Meat/Seafood Soups

Paprika	Anti-inflammatory Antioxidant	Soups Stews
Parsley	Antioxidant Antimicrobial	Seafood/ Shellfish Pasta Salads
Peppermint	Helps Stimulate Digestion Relieves GI Disorders	A Simple Snack
Rosemary	Antioxidant Anti-inflammatory Anticancer	Meat/Fish/ Poultry Dressings Sauces
Thyme	Antioxidant Inhibits Bone Resorption	Soups Dressings Marinades
Turmeric	Anticancer	South American Cuisine Curry

After cleaning out the cupboards and refrigerator of everything boxed, canned, or packaged, you may ask yourself what you are supposed to eat. Well, breakfast is the easiest and most essential meal of the day. Organic, free-range eggs are one of the healthiest foods on earth, and why not whip up a very healthy veggie omelet in the morning? If eggs aren't your thing, a fruit bowl is another favorite on my list.

For lunch, I usually do a salad that I will explain in a second. If salads do not fill you up, why not add an organic soup or a vegetable tray to go along with it? I will go into my soups in more detail, but organic lean meats are always a great choice as well. For dinner, I always grill up a lean, organic piece of meat along with steamed or raw vegetables. Of course, herbs and spices can be added to all of these meals and I highly recommend doing so.

Some other quick and easy ways to eliminate some of the processing in our kitchens is to simply make soup from scratch. Dice up some of your favorite veggies, throw them in a huge pot of organic chicken stock, add your herbs and spices, heat up, and enjoy. This is something that the whole family can enjoy for the whole week, just refrigerate and reheat. All the vegetables contain many essential vitamins and nutrients and they are also low calorie. Another health benefit I add to all my homemade soups is cut up cilantro or other herbs and spices.

Another great dinner choice is a large, bulky salad. What do I mean by bulky? Well, we need to add some substance to our salads, and this usually means a healthy protein source. This will not only make us feel full, but it will probably almost single-handedly satisfy our protein intake for the entire day (unless you're a serious body builder). Two good sources of protein are either cut-up hard-boiled egg whites or cut-up grilled chicken breast strips. Both sources of protein should be 100 percent organic. Also, we should make our salads as colorful as possible. This means getting our favorite knife out, and starting to dice up all different kinds of veggies, and changing it up as much as possible. Some of the choices I use on a regular basis are celery, carrots, broccoli, cauliflower, red and white onions, and peppers of every color. Throwing in a few cut up mushrooms will also add new taste and texture to your salad. Not only will our salads be tasteful, they will also be filling and very nutritious. If you think about it, you're basically eating a few different kinds of raw vegetables with a protein source. Raw vegetables maintain all the vitamins and nutrients that cooking may deplete. No processed food, no artificial flavors, and no preservatives. Just the way God intended us to eat. This should be your dinner two to three times every week.

I know everyone gets hungry throughout the day and evening—so what do we do for those midday and midnight cravings? One of the healthiest snacks we can have on hand is a bowl of nuts and seeds. How easy is that to have on hand when a craving occurs? This is a much healthier alternative than a sugar-loaded snack. Nuts and seeds contain many essential nutrients and oils with absolutely no sugar content. Obviously having a bowl of fruit or a veggie tray on hand is always a great idea too. The goal is to turn our unhealthy snacks and cravings into all-natural snacks and cravings.

Let's take a minute to talk about what we are sipping on all day long. Back to my number one rule, "If it wasn't here five hundred years ago, it's probably not good for us." That pretty much eliminates everything but good old H_2O. All sodas, alcohol, fruit juices, energy drinks, etc. contain useless sugars, artificial flavor and calories. In fact 56 percent of eight-year-olds down soft drinks daily, and a third of teenage boys drink at least three cans of soda pop per day.[14]

According to *The Lancet*, a British medical journal, a team of Harvard researchers presented the first evidence linking soft drink consumption to childhood obesity. They found that twelve-year-olds who drank soft drinks regularly were more likely to be overweight than those who did not.[15] Go through your kitchen right now and throw out all the soft drinks. If we can eliminate just soda immediately, your health will drastically improve. We already discussed how sugar is the number one addiction in America and the cause of most age-related degenerative diseases, but for now let's just get it out of our refrigerators and into our trash can immediately.

Another thing concerning fluids is we have to STOP drinking anything diet right now. I mean immediately!! I know this might alarm some of you coming from a "health and wellness" book, but diet drinks mean the drinks contain artificial sweeteners. Please eliminate all artificial sweeteners from your kitchen today. These include MSG, aspartame, sucralose, as well as others. Artificial sweeteners such as MSG are basically human-made chemicals that have been shown to cause a plethora of diseases and conditions including cancer. We must be very careful when cleaning out our kitchens, as a lot of these artificial sweeteners are buried in the labeling on your food. Not only are they in almost all of your diet drinks, they are also commonly found in baking goods, sweetened peanuts, health bars, meal-replacement bars, and some canned goods. Do your due diligence and examine every label in your kitchen. Trust me—these artificial sweeteners were not around five hundred years ago and they are not naturally found in nature. Statistics from the San Antonio Heart Study show that those who drink more diet soda have an increased chance they will become overweight and even obese. This twenty-five-year study was conducted at the University of Texas Health Science Center at San Antonio and was really eye-opening for those who thought they were doing their bodies a favor by drinking more diet soda than regular soda.[16] One of the theories behind this is that diet soda does not trigger your body to feel satisfied, so you will keep eating more and more calories. So not only do diet drinks contain unnatural human-made chemicals, they also might make you gain more weight than regular soda does.

I know, water is so boring, but did you know that about 65 percent of your body is water? Don't you think it is a good idea to replenish our bodies with water on a daily basis? Not to mention, water will also help eliminate and flush the toxins out of our bodies.

If we must have some flavor in our drinks, we can always enjoy a cup of green tea. Green tea is one of the most researched drinks of recent times. It is not only good for your taste buds, but also great for your health and longevity as well. According to the *Journal of American Medical Association (JAMA),* laboratory and animal studies have shown that the polyphenols in green tea may be protective against cardiovascular disease and cancer.[17] Polyphenols are chemicals in plants that have great antioxidant properties, and we need to be getting them in our diet on a daily basis. Other properties of green tea are shown to be anticancer, anti-inflammatory, antimicrobial, and probiotic. All of these great health-enhancing benefits in a simple drink. It must be the fountain of youth! Just think, instead of drinking our customary sugary drinks that contain human-made chemicals that cause disease, there is a great-tasting alternative that actually fights disease. So go clean out your fridge of all the sodas and sugary drinks and load it up with green tea and water.

Now that we have cleared out our kitchens and fridges of all the processed junk that you can find in the middle of the grocery store, we can start preparing and eating much better. Another great rule of thumb is to always shop around the perimeter of the grocery store. Feel free to buy all the **fresh produce, organic meats** and **eggs, salads, fruits** and **veggies, bottled water, green tea, herbs** and **spices, nuts, seeds,** and **berries** that your heart desires.

Patients always ask me what they are supposed to eat. I simply give them the bolded list above. It is exactly what is in my kitchen, and it is exactly what should be in all of our kitchens. Let's rid our kitchens today of all the toxins, sugars, artificial flavors, and sweeteners today and start to enjoy the health benefits that nature's foods can provide us.

Start Detoxifying Your Lifestyle Now

Cleaning out Your Kitchen

1. If it was not here five hundred years ago, get it out of your kitchen and out of your diet.

2. Eliminate all beverages except water and green tea from your refrigerator.

3. Eliminate artificial sweeteners from your kitchen.

4. Cut back the amount of processed foods in your kitchen.

5. Start buying more organic meats and produce.

6. Start reading more labels and really understanding what is in the food you are buying.

7. Shop more around the perimeter of the grocery store than inside the aisles.

8. Always have nuts, seeds, and berries on hand as snacks.

9. Start preparing more healthy meals including homemade soups and salads that contain many different vegetable sources.

10. Try to start your day off with a fruit bowl for breakfast.

Lifestyle Habit 7
Combating Emotional Stress

One the most important recommendations
in *Detoxifying our Lifestyle* is to be in a good
state of mind all the time. In my office, I call
this "giving yourself a checkup from the neck
up." Emotional stress can be defined as any
change in our normal routine that causes an
imbalance in our life. This imbalance can be
a chemical imbalance, such as an increase
in your adrenaline levels, or a physical
imbalance as well, such as tight muscles or
even a migraine. When emotional stresses
become persistent, many different symptoms
and ailments can soon follow.

People who are emotionally healthy are
in total control of their thoughts, feelings,
and behaviors from the time they wake up
in the morning until they lie down in bed at
night. Emotional stresses that we encounter

throughout the day play a major role in our physical health and wellness. From chemical imbalances and emotional sicknesses to physical ailments, a lot of what plagues America today comes down to how our bodies are able to deal with emotional stresses on a daily basis.

I am not going to sit here and lie to you and say that I can rid your life of stress, but I will tell you that if you follow a lot of the dietary recommendations that have already been laid out in this book, your body will be in a much better position to deal with daily stresses. Just take a look at the chart on the next page to see all the ailments that have been linked to emotional stress. With a few simple exercises and stress-reducing habits that we can do on a daily basis, we can put ourselves, our minds, and our tension levels at ease. It takes only a few minutes a day, but it can produce decades of healthier years to enjoy. After all, life is such a great adventure—there is no reason not to enjoy it for as long as possible.

Ailments linked to excessive emotional stress

*Headaches
*Backaches
*Mood swings
*Restlessness and inability to fall asleep
*Diarrhea or constipation
*Muscle stiffness
*Muscle aches and pains
*Chest pain
*Memory problems
*Dizziness
*Inability to concentrate
*Anxiousness
*Teeth grinding
*Skin breakouts
*Weakened immune system with chronic colds/flu
*Feeling overwhelmed
*Double vision
*Chronic migraines
*Rapid heartbeat
*Increased blood pressure
*Accelerated aging process

One of the most crucial problems that stress can cause is the effect it has on weakening our immune systems. Our immune systems play such a vital role in health, wellness, and longevity. We have already talked about how different foods and nutrients can either strengthen or weaken our immunity, but thoughts, feelings, and emotions can also strengthen or weaken our immune system. Negative emotional stress definitely interferes with the immune system in a negative way and weakens the body's natural line of defense. On the other side of the coin, positive emotional stress will definitely strengthen our body and immune system. Cancer survivors often talk about how they beat cancer with a positive attitude and laughter. It has also been shown that laughter actually increases our immune cells and decreases stress, tension, and muscle spasm. I think it's time to get a regular seat at the local comedy club.

White blood cells are our bodies' immune cells; these are the cells that are constantly fighting off infection and toxins within us. In a study reported in the medical journal *Health Psychology*, twenty-five stressed-out parents were evaluated. These twenty-five parents were stressed because their children were diagnosed with cancer. I am pretty sure any parent would be stressed in this scenario. The study evaluated the white blood cells of the twenty-five stressed parents. They found that the white blood cells of the stressed parents were less responsive than those of parents of healthy children. The study proved emotional stresses actually cause a physical response in the body, and these parents were more likely to have problems with their immune systems and health. It then showed that stressed parents who were reported to have a lot of support from family members had immune responses similar to those of the nonstressed parents.[18] I think it's just amazing how our outside emotional stresses affect our bodies, all the way down to the cellular level.

This is the basis for different types of alternative medicines such as chiropractic and acupuncture. Techniques like these alternative treatments work all the way down to the cellular level. In fact, it has been shown that regular chiropractic adjustments can increase your white blood cell count as well as naturally lower your blood pressure. All this with no negative side effects that drugs can cause. We should definitely make sure chiropractors, acupuncturists, and massage therapists are part of our health and wellness team that we see on a regular basis.

There are many other things we can be doing on a daily basis that will help our body deal with life's stresses. One of the very first things we can do every morning is to start our day off by reading or reciting affirmations. Positive affirmations can put us at ease, get us in a positive mind-set to start our day, and even bring us whatever we desire. People have used daily affirmations to help them lose weight, gain prosperity, and get job promotions. These success stories are believed to work through affirmations by continually telling our subconscious mind what to believe. The ability to control our very own subconscious mind can be very powerful, and guide us in the right direction to always have a positive attitude, which in turn will greatly reduce our emotional stress level.

If we start our day off on the wrong foot, it seems like the whole day snowballs into negative events, and unpleasant circumstances just keep arising. On the other hand, if we get off on the right foot, it can make for a very happy and successful day. Do you know a person who just seems lucky all the time? We must understand that luck begins with belief, and with belief, anything is possible. Daily affirmations will put our subconscious mind and us in a positive mode every morning. Trust me—good things will begin to happen. For some people, it's going take longer than for others because you're not going to really believe what you're saying, but stick with the affirmations every morning and soon enough your "luck" will start to shift. If you are new to affirmations, take a look at the sample affirmations on the next page. You can either come up with your own or search for affirmations that you believe will help you the most. Most importantly, be consistent with them every morning, and really feel and recite the affirmations with emotion.

Daily Affirmation Samples

Tomorrow will be the best day possible. Great and exciting things will happen to me tomorrow. My mind, body, and soul will experience a great day. I will feel energized, motivated, and will be able to accomplish all my goals tomorrow. An amazing day awaits me.

Amazing opportunities await me every day. I am filled with good luck. I appreciate all the amazing things that happen to me each and every day. Good things and good people always show up in my life. I am grateful for all the goodness today is about to bring me.

My mind and body are very powerful. I use my gifts to attract abundance and goodness to me every day. I am grateful for having the health, wealth, friendship, and all abundances in my life. I will use my gifts today to help others, knowing that by helping others, I am also helping myself.

As I sleep tonight, I allow my mind, body, and soul to relax and rejuvenate. Tonight will bring me great sleep and relaxation. I grow stronger and healthier with each passing moment tonight. I am the embodiment of health and abundance.

Food is for my health and well-being. I will eat only that which is healthy and organic today. I trust that my body will be at its ideal weight. I make great choices for health and longevity. I will thoroughly enjoy my workout today, as I know it will help me.

Detoxify Your Lifestyle Exercise – How Stressed Am I?

1. I have a hard time falling asleep at night.
A. Not at all
B. Rarely
C. Sometimes
D. Always

2. My mind is racing about everything I have to do as soon as I wake up.
A. Not at all
B. Rarely
C. Sometimes
D. Always

3. I feel tired physically and emotionally throughout the day.
A. Not at all
B. Rarely
C. Sometimes
D. Always

4. I am constantly concerned about my financial situation.
A. Not at all
B. Rarely
C. Sometimes
D. Always

5. I believe I have control over my success or failure.

A. 100 percent of the time.

B. Sometimes

C. Rarely

D. It seems out of my control.

6. I can confide in my significant other about anything.

A. Yes

B. Most anything

C. Not really

D. I keep a lot to myself.

7. I work so much that my outside relationships are suffering.

A. Not at all.

B. I try to keep in touch.

C. I find it hard to keep in touch.

D. Yes

8. I turn to comfort food or alcohol when stressed.

A. Not at all.

B. Rarely

C. Sometimes

D. Almost always.

9. When presented with a difficult task, I hit it head-on and try to accomplish it immediately.

A. Yes – 100 percent.
B. Most of the time.
C. I get frustrated.
D. I completely break down.

10. Every winter I catch a cold or flu at least once.

A. Not at all.
B. Rarely
C. Sometimes
D. Most likely

Now add up your score with: A=1, B=2, C=3, D=4

*10–18 – You are doing fairly well with your stress levels, but there is always room for improvement.

*19–26 – You need a little work with your stress levels. Be sure to read about our stress-reducing habits you can incorporate into your life.

*27–33 – Your stress levels are fairly high and most likely affecting your health, wellness, and longevity. Be sure to incorporate our stress-reducing habits and make some lifestyle changes in order to cope with your stresses.

*34–40 – Outside stresses are controlling your life and affecting your health. It is time to make some serious changes immediately or your health, wellness, and longevity will be greatly affected.

Another great tool to help relieve our daily stresses is yoga. Yoga has been around for many years and it works really well. By definition, yoga is the art of unifying the mind, body, and soul. A session of yoga will leave us feeling at peace with ourselves because of the natural realignment of our body and mind. For beginners, yoga will help us breathe easier and relax our body. As we get more advanced in the art of yoga, we will start to experience spiritual awakening and a totally relaxed state of mind. Through continued yoga, we will be able to control our emotions and stresses much better throughout our day. We will even be able to take a five-minute break out of our day for a quick session of yoga. This will help lower our blood pressure and help our muscles relax during the grind of our daily schedules. It will also help us take a step back and breathe, which will help reoxygenate our body. There are many ways we can participate in yoga nowadays. We can either go to our local health club and take classes from teachers, or we can simply purchase a yoga DVD and practice yoga in the comfort of our own home. There is nothing better than a good yoga session to start our day off on the right foot.

Benefits of Yoga

Increases flexibility
Improves respiration
Lubricates joints/ligaments/tendons
Helps relax the mind and body
Detoxifies the body
Promotes circulatory health
Tones muscles
Helps athletic performance

If yoga doesn't seem like your thing, simply do five to ten minutes of stretching each morning or evening. Stretching isn't just for getting warmed up before an athletic competition. We can all benefit from a few minutes of stretching each day. Stretching on a regular basis will also help us deal with our daily stresses. Stretching will help keep joints nice and lubricated; it will keep ligaments and tendons loose and keep our muscles from becoming knotted up. It will also help clear our head of negative emotions, thoughts, and stresses.

One of the first places stress attacks is our neck and upper shoulder muscles, also known as our trapezius muscles. As a chiropractor, almost every patient I see can use some work in his or her neck and trapezius area. It is just where most of us hold our stress. These muscles become very knotted and can definitely cause a lot of different health problems. I have seen knotted muscles in the neck and trapezius cause headaches, migraines, vertigo, carpal tunnel syndrome, eye problems, TMJ disorders, and chronic ear and throat infections in children. As we age, these muscles seem to become increasingly tight and more knotted up. Daily stretching can keep these stressed muscles from getting out of control and causing health issues. It is as easy as that, five to ten minutes a day of stretching can greatly reduce some common health issues that I treat every day. Stretching can easily be done while showering in the morning, during our lunch break, or while watching our favorite show in the evening. There is really no excuse not to stretch on a daily basis.

Benefits of Stretching

Increases your range of motion
Calms breathing
Keeps muscles nice and loose
Helps blood flow
Helps detoxify the body
Keeps joints lubricated
Increases energy levels
Increases flexibility
Relieves stress
Increases coordination
Improves posture

Another great five-minute habit that can help with daily stress is deep breathing. Think about it, we can live about a month without food and about a week without water; take a guess how long we can survive without breathing. Yeah, pretty easy question. Something this essential to our health probably deserves a little more attention from us.

Throughout our daily lives, our breaths can become shallow and stagnant. Taking just one minute to ourselves throughout our busy day can help relax muscles, increase circulation, relieve unwanted tension, and lower our blood pressure.

Breathing will also get our lymphatic system running properly. Think of the lymph system as our body's waste management system. Lymph vessels run throughout the entire body and form a drainage system to get rid of all the waste products that are produced in our body through the thousands of chemical reactions that occur every day. There are actually more lymph vessels in our body than blood vessels. When our lymph system is not clean and clear, the body cannot detoxify properly, or get rid of all the waste products. When the waste products are stuck in our body, problems start to arise. Are you catching on to how important this circuitry is? Unfortunately, we don't hear a lot about our lymphatic system unless someone is diagnosed with cancer. A lot of different types of cancers spread through the lymph vessels. We should be trying to keep our lymph system clean, clear, and running properly if we want to be healthy. Deep breathing and exercise will keep our lymph fluid running properly throughout the body and it will not become stagnant. When the lymphatic system is moving properly, the body has a very good chance of detoxifying itself. While deep breathing will keep everything clean and clear inside, we will also be removing stress in the meantime.

A good way to practice deep breathing is to exhale twice as long as you inhale, with a four-second pause in between. For example, take a deep inhale for six seconds, pause for four seconds, and exhale very slowly for twelve seconds.

Inhale – six seconds
Pause – four seconds
Exhale – twelve seconds

Repeat this for two to three minutes throughout the day. It would not be hard at all to do this at the top of the hour at the office throughout the day. The benefits will be well worth it.

Probably the very best way to get ourselves out of a rut and relieve our emotional stresses is to show and feel gratitude. When we are bombarded with stress every single day, it starts to put us in a negative attitude, and makes a lot of us feel as if the world is against us. Gratitude is a very positive emotion (maybe the most positive emotion) about a benefit that one receives. The power of gratitude is very hard to grasp for some people. With practice, gratitude will show us clarity from confusion in an unbalanced life. Research has shown this very powerful feeling is beneficial to our emotional well-being. In my practice, I have noticed that those who show me more gratitude tend to be much happier in their own lives.

Many wealth experts say that wealth equals gratitude. By the "Law of Attraction," if we want to increase our wealth, we should really focus on being more grateful. The wealth will soon follow. I believe we can substitute "health" for "wealth" in this scenario. If we want to be healthier, focus on what we are grateful for and the health benefits will soon follow. For example, if you have chronic migraines, much of your focus and life will revolve around these migraines. You will always wonder if today you are going to get one. What happens if you get one at work? How will you take care of your kids? How are you supposed to get everything done if you get a migraine today? As you can see, the whole day is consumed about worrying and focusing on the migraine. Instead, we should focus on gratitude for other parts of our life that are great. Why not show thanks for your family, friends, home, the food on your table, your great job, your supporting spouse, etc. Do you get the picture? Please do not let the negative parts of your life consume your thoughts. It will just spark more negativity, and in this case, more migraines.

In my practice, I treat a lot of high school- and college-age children who have problems with depression, anxiety, anger, ADHD, and so on. At this age, a lot of these types of children are revolting against their parents. You know, it's just that time in their lives. We were all teenagers at one point. One of the first practices I do with this type of patient is send them home and have them write down, on paper, fifty things they are thankful for. Parents are continually telling me what a great exercise this is for their children. Of course, they always write how thankful they are for their family and parents. I can then reiterate over and over how appreciative they should be for having a loving family and parents. This is a real eye-opener for these kids, and they start to see their family life in a different light, and soon their depressive-anxiety or anger issues dramatically decline.

The point is we can all attest to getting in a rut throughout our busy lives, but sitting down and really thinking about how thankful we should be for our blessings will really help combat whatever emotional stress we happen to be going through at any particular time. I start every morning off with affirmations that actually contain many statements about being grateful. When we really practice this exercise and do it consistently, we will really start to have the feelings and emotions of the power of gratitude. It is one thing to just say "I am thankful for_____," but you really have to have the feeling behind it. Check out the next page for some sample affirmations of this emotion.

Grateful Affirmations

*I am grateful and thankful for all goodness
God has given me.
*I give thanks daily for blessings that flow into
my life.
*I am grateful for my health.
*I am grateful for losing weight on my continuing
journey to health, wellness, and longevity.
*I am grateful for my beautiful family.
*I am grateful for my fulfilling and prosperous job.
*I am grateful to have the freedom to live the life
of my dreams.
*I am grateful for my wide array of friends and
business associates.
*I am thankful for my beautiful home.
*I know gratitude is a daily choice and I choose to
be grateful.
*I am grateful for my faith.

Once again, I cannot promise that we can rid all of the emotional stress life throws at us. I think it's just impossible. We can, however, train our minds, bodies, and souls to better cope with our daily stresses, and therefore keep our bodies much, much stronger. Every day, patients walk into my office with a particular ache or pain and they go on to tell me exactly how it happened. They try to pinpoint it to the exact moment. "I was just getting out of my car when my back went out." Well, you get out of your car fifty times per week. What was different about this particular time? I constantly have to reiterate that it's not one exact point in time. It is a buildup of all the stresses, and finally the body cannot take any more, and it breaks down. This is a hard concept for a lot of people to really understand. Yes, we do want to eliminate as many outside stresses as possible, but more importantly take on a few habits that will help our bodies, minds, and spirits deal with the stresses for many years to come. There are many quick and easy things we can do on a daily basis to help calm our nerves, muscles, and blood pressure. It's just like brushing our teeth though; we must do it a couple of times every single day. Do not wait until you wake up one day and don't recognize yourself in the mirror; start to combat your stresses today and slow down the aging process. You will thank yourself later.

Start Detoxifying Your Lifestyle Now

1. Start each and every morning off with positive affirmations.

2. Write down on paper where your emotional stress comes from and learn to recognize it.

3. Make sure you are laughing every single day!!

4. Go to sleep at the same time every night and wake up at the same time every morning.

5. Use yoga on a regular basis to combat stress!

6. Visit your chiropractor and massage therapist regularly!

7. Stop for a few minutes each day and take some deep breaths.

8. Start to stretch first thing in the morning and before bed.

9. Write down a list of fifty things that you are thankful for, and make sure you show gratitude each day.

10. Smile!

Lifestyle Habit 8
Specific Exercise

So we all know that exercise is very, very good for us. It is absolutely something that we need to be doing every single day. Of course, we all know by now the benefits of exercise. It will help our hearts and arteries, keep us looking good in our bathing suits, and fill us with energy. What a lot of us do not know, most likely, is the best specific types of exercise that will give us the most benefits for our health, wellness, and longevity. We will also talk about different types of exercise programs that we should stay away from because they might actually do more harm than good. As always, we will relate exercise back to our ancestors and how they got their exercise many years ago. Trust me—they were not out running marathons and very long distances that were detrimental to their body.

So what did our ancestors do for exercise? Most of them were hunters and gatherers. This type of lifestyle demanded a lot of physical exertion and movement. Their daily exercise consisted of walking and running in search of food. They would walk for a while, climb, swim, and sprint after wild animals, such as buffaloes. If you asked yourself what type of exercise I just explained, it can be classified as cross-training exercise. Studies of these hunters and gathers show very little to no signs of cardiovascular disease,[19] one of the top killers, if not the top killer, in America today. This can be attributed not only to their daily types of exercise, but also to their diet, which was free of sugars, carbohydrates, and processed grains.

As a human population, we have evolved immensely from our hunting and gathering days, but since genetics takes so many years to evolve, we should still be exercising just like we did many years ago. Back then, their very livelihood could depend on being able to sprint away from a predator or sprint toward an animal for the kill. If you don't get the kill, you simply do not eat that day. It was a very high-intensity type of training back then. Of course, we do not have to worry about sprinting for our lives anymore, but our exercise regimes should really reflect the lives of our ancestors. They should consist of high-intensity sprint workouts and resistance exercises. We should also be looking for new challenges and new types of exercise in order to keep our bodies challenged. If we were truly hunters and gatherers, we would not be doing the exact same movements and physical exercises day in and day out. So what makes us think using the same machines at your local health club every Monday, Wednesday, and Friday would be beneficial? We definitely need to keep mixing things up, but overall, they should be sprint or interval exercises coupled with resistance training. We will get more in depth about the types of exercises later in this chapter, but first I have to tell you a story of the first marathon ever run. In no way, do I believe running long distances is very good for our long-term health, and the very first marathon in history helps support my thoughts on this subject.

Being a Greek-American, and growing up in a Greek household, I remember hearing the story of the very first marathon at a young age. The story takes place in the fifth century BC. The Persians and the Greeks were at war. The Persians were known for their dominance and were very powerful in this era. The

Greeks, on the other hand, consisted of many small city-states, and were not as powerful as their counterparts, the Persians. Athens eventually became the most powerful city in Greece, and became the capital of Greece. During these years, the Persian Empire was rapidly expanding over the Mediterranean Sea and into Greece. They had been moving toward Athens in hopes of conquering the Greek Empire. They were 26.2 miles away from Athens in a small city called Marathon. The Greek army was outnumbered about four to one, but initiated a surprise attack on the Persians. At the end of the day, sixty-four hundred Persian bodies lay dead on the field. A Greek soldier named Phidippides was called upon to run from the battle of Marathon to Athens to report the news of victory. Phidippides rose to the challenge and ran his heart out to the city of Athens, which was exactly 26.2 miles away. This is now known as the first marathon in history. Phidippides pushed himself very hard on his trek back to Athens. The story goes that he ran the 26.2 miles in under three hours. Top marathon runners today run a marathon in around two hours. So he ran the very first marathon in an extremely impressive time without any previous marathon or distance training.

Phidippides delivered the message that the Greek army had beaten the Persians, then fell over and died. We know that exercise is very, very good for us, but we need to know what types of exercise are good for our bodies, and what types of exercises are actually detrimental to our health.

As humans, we are not meant to run or exercise for long distances. The prestigious medical journal, *Circulation*, did a study on Boston marathon runners. The study tested sixty runners in the 2004 and 2005 Boston marathons. They did pre and post heart studies, such as echocardiographs, on the runners. The study concluded that completion of a marathon is associated with correlative biochemical and echocardiograph evidence of cardiac dysfunction and injury, and this risk is increased in those participants with less training.[20] Simply put, running twenty-six miles causes irreversible damage to our heart. Again, the human body is not meant to do this. By no means am I advocating *not* exercising, but I do want to stress the proper types of exercise that will benefit us the most for our own health, wellness, and longevity. Another great example of this point is the great Jim Fixx. Jim Fixx was an American icon among marathon runners. He was the author of the best-selling 1977 book, *The Complete Book of Running*. He moved millions of Americans to get off their butts and start exercising. Of course, he was pushing Americans to run and jog long distances. I commend him for his efforts to get us off our butts and moving. Jim Fixx, an avid long-distance runner, died of a heart attack at the age of fifty-two years young. Once again, there are better ways to get our daily exercise in.

Besides taking a toll on our hearts, long-distance training also places a huge burden on our joints—specifically our ankles, knees, and hip joints. I have come across many long-distance runners in my practice that have severe arthritis in these joints and even total joint replacements at the young ages of forty, fifty, and sixty years old. The daily wear and tear on these joints from hitting the pavement for long distances over the years takes a major toll on the cartilage within the joints. The cartilage in our joints acts as a shock absorber between our bones. Every step we take wears down those shock absorbers a little more and a little more. So if we are running long distances, especially on the pavement for many years, we will wear down those shock absorbers much more quickly and speed up the arthritis process. That is why I see many middle-aged patients, with worn-down joints such as hips and knees. Sometimes, the only option is to get an artificial joint. The moral of the story is that the body is supposed to be able to handle physical exertion and physical exercise. When we perform an activity over and over again that the body is not supposed to be doing in the first place, it is going to cause problems. Maybe not right away, but eventually we will experience side effects. If we do more specific interval-type training, the joints of our bodies will be able to hold up and perform pain free at age one hundred. Let's just do the activities that we are supposed to do and we will all be better off for it. Always remember that too much exercise might be just as bad as not enough. We need to find the happy medium of the proper amount of exercise as well as the right types of exercise.

Benefits of Proper Exercise

Helps keep arteries clear
Increases lung capacity
Increases blood flow
Helps detoxify the body
Keeps spine and joints loose and lubricated
Helps clean out the lymphatic system
Helps keep you feeling and looking young
Helps maintain optimal body weight
Can increase your HDL (good) cholesterol
Keeps blood pressure in optimal ranges
Helps with sleep problems
Is a great stress-reducing activity
Helps with our mental state

Detoxify Your Lifestyle Exercise Quiz

1. How many days per week do you do at least thirty minutes of cardiovascular exercise?

A. 0-2

B. 3-4

C. 5-6

D. 7 or more

2. How many days/week do you do at least thirty minutes of strength (resistance) training?

A. 0-2

B. 3-4

C. 5-6

D. 7 or more

3. Is it a struggle for you to get up and exercise every day?

A. always

B. most of the time

C. not usually

D. never

4. When exercising, do you always work up a good sweat?

A. never

B. sometimes

C. most of the time

D. always

5. Do your entertainment activities consist of physical activities or sedentary activities?

A. always sedentary

B. mostly sedentary

C. mostly physical

D. always physical

6. What best describes you?

A. I don't know how to reach my goals.

B. I can't stick with a program.

C. I know what to do, but I'm not where I want to be.

D. I currently exercise regularly, but need a challenge both physically and mentally.

7. What resources for exercise do you have available to you?

A. none

B. I have a few weights at home.

C. I have a gym membership.

D. I have a personal strength and conditioning coach.

8. I stretch before and after exercise.

A. I never stretch

B. only before

C. only after workout

D. I always stretch before and after my workout.

9. When starting a new exercise program I usually:

A. never follow through more than a week
B. always make excuses and miss workouts
C. quit after one month because of boredom
D. always follow through the entire program

10. When I think about exercise, I think about:

A. how much I dislike exercise
B. how hard it will be
C. trying to make excuses why I can't exercise today
D. how good I will feel after my workout

Now add up your score with: A=1, B=2, C=3, D=4

*10-16 – You need to get a new outlook on your physical exercise levels, really commit to an exercise regime, and understand how important exercise is for your overall health.

*17-23 – You need to recommit to your exercise levels, get a brand new program, and stick with it for an extended amount of time.

*24-30 – Your exercise levels are doing fairly well, but continue to read and learn new types of exercise programs, set new goals for yourself, and take your exercise to a whole new level this year.

*31-40 – You are doing great as far as exercise is concerned. Keep it up. What you can do is keep making new goals for yourself and continue to reach new heights as far as physical exercise is concerned.

Now that we have gone over how our ancestors got their "exercise" many years ago, let's dig in and really discover what we should be doing today. I really don't want us sprinting after buffalo and killing them with our swords or spears. We have all watched the Olympics at some point in our lives. I want to compare a one-hundred-yard sprinter to a long-distance runner. The sprinters are always very lean, muscular, and look very healthy. We can see every muscle fiber in their bodies, as they have no body fat—basically everything we want to look like when bikini season rolls around. The long-distance runners look skinny as well, but they look like an unhealthy skinny. They usually look frail, their eyes are sunken in, they look malnourished, and just do not look like the healthiest people overall. The difference between these two types of athletes is that one is exercising just like the human body is supposed to exercise and the other is actually causing harm to his or her body with an exercise regime.

Let's dig a little deeper into these two different kinds of training. The long-distance trainer wakes up every morning, puts on running shoes, and hits the open road. The runner might spend an hour or more for a morning run and then at night do it all over again. This is both unhealthy and detrimental to health. First of all, every time we exercise we are creating free radicals in our body. Remember, free radicals are not good and actually cause things like cancer and heart disease. Now, exercise is still good, but every type of exercise does and will cause the production of free radicals inside our bodies. That is why there are different types of exercise that are good and other types of exercise that actually do more harm than good. When we are performing long-distance exercise and putting in mile after mile, our bodies produce an enormous amount of free radicals. It is almost as if our bodies are in survival mode when we have an exercise regime like this. Year after year and mile after mile, we are putting a lot more pressure on our bodies. I have treated many baby boomers who have been running long distances for years. Many have run year after year for forty to fifty years. All of these patients are now coming in with knee, hip, ankle, and low back pain caused by the pressure of running for all those years. Can you imagine the pounding these joints have taken over the decades? I cannot even help many of these patients and have to refer them out for knee and hip replacements. Trust me—we all want our own knee and hip joints, not some artificial stainless steel joint. These human-made artificial joints will never be as good as the ones our parents gave us.

I am not saying that these people made a huge mistake by wanting to run and exercise all their lives. I commend them for doing so, but they need to stop their way of training right now and get to a more interval-based training. We just didn't know years ago that there were more beneficial types of training out there for us. A few decades ago, running long distance was the thing to do, and we thought it was the fountain of youth. Now, however, research has caught up with us, and we realize there is a better way. Remember, at one point in time, we also didn't know that cigarettes were bad for us. It is OK that the "jogging fad" hit America. It at least made us start thinking about exercise. Now, we need to take it a step further, and really get specific about exercise and start a program that will best serve our bodies.

This takes us to interval training, or sprint training. This is how our Olympic sprinters have been training for years, and it is exactly how the hunters and gatherers lived their daily lives many years ago. We are not going to need an expensive trainer or a high-tech stopwatch to start our interval training program. As a matter of fact, we will not need anything that we do not have right now. All we really need is a mind-set that we are going to switch up how we perform our daily exercises. Most treadmills, bikes, and elliptical machines already have an interval regime programmed into them. We all know the one—when we go really hard for one minute, then relax for a couple minutes, and keep repeating that sequence for twenty to twenty-five minutes. This type of training is actually going to save a lot of distance runners many hours per week, and you'll definitely see the results both physically and mentally. Our hearts, lungs, and joints are also going to reap the benefits.

Along with the interval-type cardio training, the second aspect of this type of training is resistance training. We need to be working our muscles. I don't care how we do it, but all the muscles of our body need to be challenged. Every time a muscle is worked, it burns up glucose. This means less glucose floating around in our bloodstream wreaking havoc on all our bodies' processes. In Chapter 3, we discovered how to decrease the amount of sugar we put in our mouths or even completely eliminate it altogether, and now we know how to get rid of sugar once it is in our bloodstreams. If we're going to put it in our bodies through our diets, we must burn it up through exercise.

By now you should realize I am pretty blunt about giving health and lifestyle advice. I am going to come right out and say we need to be exercising every single day. I am not going to sugarcoat it and tell you that three times per week is sufficient. It is not. There are seven days in a week, so let's exercise seven days. Do you brush your teeth only three days a week? That's what I thought. Just make it a habit, and do the right amount of exercise every day. In my office, we do not take excuses such as I don't have enough time. I am asking for only twenty to forty minutes a day. If you can't make twenty to forty minutes a day for your health, I am not sure how you even made it to this chapter, but I have faith that you will start to make that twenty to forty minutes per day consistently for the rest of your life. If a patient tells me, he or she doesn't have time and refuses to make twenty to forty minutes a day, I will simply tell the person that he or she doesn't have time for health, wellness, and longevity. Please come back when you have time and want to commit to getting your health and wellness where it needs to be. I cannot tell you enough how important exercise is for each and every one of us. We all must realize that without our health, we are nothing.

Now, to get more specific on what we need to be doing. The forty minutes is broken down into twenty minutes of interval cardio exercise and twenty minutes of resistance exercise. For the interval cardio exercise, we can pretty much do any type of cardiovascular exercise we want. Although, we should always be switching it up all the time. I personally like swimming, biking, cross-country skiing or elliptical machines, sprinting, hill sprints, and steps. Go as fast and strong as you can for one minute, and then a very slow recovery pace for one minute and thirty seconds. This alternating type of interval cardio training has existed for years, but new findings and studies now show how much better this type of exercise is for us. It will not only improve our cardiovascular health, but it will tap into our natural fat-burning capabilities as well. New evidence also shows that interval training protects us against heart attacks much better than endurance running. In our strong phase, we want to really be working at 100 percent capacity. This means we should not able to talk to our training partner because we are breathing too hard. In our recover phase, we want to be at around 30 percent maximum capacity, and by the end of the recovery phase we should have our breath back.

As far as strength or resistance training goes, this makes up the second twenty minutes of our daily exercise. I would say the majority of people hit the gym and use conventional weight training for this aspect of their exercise program, or maybe you have a weight set at home. Either way is great, but it doesn't have to be conventional weight training. As long as muscles are getting pushed to a level that makes them really work, that is sufficient. We can get this through various types of exercise. Some people like core exercises such as doing a Swiss ball routine. Others like rock climbing, which is definitely a resistance type of exercise. Some people stay away from the weight room and simply do push-ups, pull-ups, and lunges. All of these are completely fine. Just remember we are working muscle and in turn burning glucose. We can use our favorite machines at our local gym, while other people enjoy dumbbells and free weights. People get way too caught up in how to strength train. Just get in the gym and push some weight around. Unless we are trying out for the next Mr. Olympia or want to look like Arnold

Schwarzenegger, resistance training does not have to be an exact science. The old saying "use it or lose it" is still very true today. We must use those muscles every single day, and, of course, I do not want us in the gym for hours and hours. A quick twenty to thirty minutes is sufficient as long as we make a habit of it every single day. We cannot skip a few days and then spend four hours in the gym on Saturday. The body doesn't work that way. We must give it a little time every day. As I said, I don't take the excuse that you can't give yourself forty minutes a day for your health, wellness, and longevity.

Stay away from the long three- to four-mile jogs outside and the easy thirty- to forty-five-minute jaunts on the elliptical machine; start moving toward shorter workouts with higher intensity, and your body is going to respond like it never has before. Every time I walk into my local health club, I cringe when I see the whole line of treadmills with people either walking or jogging at a low-intensity pace. I just want to kick them in high gear and into interval training. Cut the amount of time spent at the gym in half, and see twice the results. Not only will you see the results within your body, but your body will also reap the longevity benefits. With the combination of interval training and resistance training, we will burn more calories, lose more fat, start to see lean muscle tissue that is hidden right now, and improve cardiovascular health tremendously. Almost too good to be true. All this while spending less time at the gym. It is that easy. I just do not understand why millions of people are spending too much time at the gym and not getting tremendous health benefits out of it. I don't want us to think that this is easy or "social time" at the gym. Trust me—you are going to be working much harder than you have been. Your heart rate will be higher and you will be breathing much more rapidly than your normal routine. The only difference is that you will decrease the amount of time you spend at the gym. Below is a sample of interval "hill sprints" that you can use. Plugging in a treadmill, bike, or stair stepper are definitely other great exercises, but I want you to get the idea of the time frame and intensity. The workout is started and finished with a three- to five-minute slight jog and stretching.

Week	Reps	Work	Recovery	Total workout time
1	6	60-sec. hill sprint	walk-back (2 mins)	18 minutes
2	8	60-sec. hill sprint	walk back (2 mins)	24 minutes
3	10	60-sec hill sprint	walk back (1.5 mins)	25 minutes
4	10	45-sec. hill sprint	walk back (1.5 min)	22.5 minutes

So this shows the general idea of how we can start doing interval training. Total workout time goes from eighteen minutes to twenty-two and a half minutes, but rather than just going out for a nice little jog for twenty-five minutes, we are going really hard with enough rest to recover. On a lot of the treadmills and other cardio machines now, we can actually program this type of workout into the menu. This makes it really easy to jump on the machine and start your interval routine at the gym. If you're an outside runner or biker, just find a location where you'll be doing your intervals and you are ready to go.

Detoxify Your Lifestyle Now

1. Set aside a time for exercise each and every day!!

2. Write out an exercise program on paper that you will follow.

3. Start an exercise journal so you can keep track of your progress.

4. If you are a long-distance exerciser, switch to interval or circuit training.

5. Incorporate resistance training into your exercise.

6. Stretch before and after every exercise session.

7. Incorporate more physical activities into your lifestyle such as biking, climbing, and skiing, instead of sitting on your couch and watching movies.

8. Make sure you are working out hard enough to sweat!!

9. Make working out FUN—invite friends and family along for the ride!

Lifestyle Habit 9
Detoxifying Teammates

Let's be honest; it is much easier to do something as a team than accomplish it by ourselves. That is why this chapter is dedicated to showing us some people who are right at home in our very own communities who will help us *detoxify our lifestyle*. This is a list of wellness experts we need to be in contact with on a regular basis for the rest of our lives if we want to reach ultimate health and wellness. Reaching our health goals has a lot to do with continued learning, as does having a wellness team around us that will help keep us motivated, and on the right path. These wellness professionals will also help us succeed in reaching our goals, making new goals to achieve, and taking our lifestyles to the next level.

After this chapter, I want you to sit down and do some homework. Start to compile a list of wellness professionals in your community that you can start using. This chapter will show us who and why we need these people in our lives. We will see some of them very often and see others maybe just a couple of times a year. Overall, these are the types of people we need for the rest of our lives in order to have long lives of health and wellness! After you compile a list of your local health and wellness experts, go ahead and call them and give them a mini interview to make sure they fit what you want, and that you feel comfortable with them. After all, they are here for you, and you should definitely have a good bond with them and feel motivated by them.

Detoxify Your Lifestyle Questionnaire

1. How regularly do you receive a chiropractic wellness adjustment?

A. once/week

B. 1x/month

C. 3-4x/year

D. only go when I am in pain

2. How often do you get a full body massage?

A. once/week

B. 1x/month

C. 3-4x/year

D. only go when I am in pain

3. How often do you partake in a yoga/Pilates (or similar) class?

A. once/week

B. 1x/month

C. 3-4x/year

D. very rarely to never

4. How often do you seek professional advice on your health and wellness?

A. once/week

B. 1x/month

C. 3-4x/year

D. very rarely to never

5. How often do you go to your physician for a regular checkup including blood work and a nutritional exam?

A. every 6 months

B. every year

C. I have only a few times in my lifetime

D. I believe I have no need to at this point

6. How often do you get nutritional advice from a certified nutritionist?

A. every 3-6 months

B. once per year

C. I have only once or twice in my lifetime

D. I believe I have no need to at this point

7. How often do you see an acupuncturist?

A. once per week

B. 1x/month

C. 3-4x per year

D. only go when I am in pain

8. How often do you go to the spa for a day of relaxation?

A. once per week

B. 1x/month

C. 3-4x per year

D. only go when I am stressed

9. How often do you read self-help books about your wellness?

A. once per week
B. 1x/month
C. 3-4x per year
D. very rarely or never

10. How would you rate your overall commitment to yourself as far as your health, wellness, and longevity are concerned?

A. extremely committed
B. somewhat committed
C. not very committed at all
D. I do not care about my health, wellness, and longevity

Now add up your score with A=4, B=3, C=2, D=1

*10-17 – You need to read and study *Detoxify Your Lifestyle* and commit to getting the right type of wellness professionals in your life.

*18-24 – You need to start looking for and including wellness professionals in your life on a regular basis.

*25-32 – You currently do many wellness activities that will help keep your body detoxified and feeling younger; read further to add a few more wellness activities to your life.

*33-40 – You currently do many wellness activities and are on your way to health, wellness, and longevity. Keep up the good work and keep learning about how to stay young and enjoy life!

Chiropractic

Chiropractic might be the biggest misconception in America's health care today. Most people believe the art of chiropractic is based on back pain, headaches, neck pain, etc. This is far from the truth. As a matter of fact, chiropractic really has absolutely nothing to do with symptoms. It is actually the science, art, and philosophy of removing nerve pressure from the body. I am sorry to say that we all have nerve pressure on our spines and nervous systems. Think of nerve pressure as stress on the spine and nervous system.

No matter how old we may be, what daily activities we do, what our occupations are, or how good or bad our diets are, we all have stress on our nervous system. No ifs, ands, or buts about it. As we have already learned throughout this book, we are bombarded with stresses and toxins on a daily (or hourly) basis. We just can't avoid them all, but what we can do is take on habits that help eliminate the stresses and toxins from our bodies. Chiropractic is one of those habits that we need to practice on a regular basis to help keep our body de-stressed and detoxified.

Here is a little bit more about the nervous system and just how vital it is to our health, wellness, and longevity. The nervous system is the master control center of every function of the body. The nervous system is made up of the brain, spinal cord, and all the thousands of nerves that run throughout the body. Picture it as a circuit board with all the connections and wires intertwined. If one of the connections is broken, the information can't get from point A to point B, and then the circuit does not carry out its job.

This is essentially how the body works. The brain is constantly sending signals down the spinal cord and out through an intertwined network of nerves until it reaches its destination point and controls some type of function in the body. For example, every second of life, the brain is sending a signal to the heart, and those signals tell the heart to beat over and over and over. What do you think happens if that signal doesn't get from the brain to the heart? You are out of luck. Are you now realizing why the nervous system is so important?

Again, all of us have some pressure on our nerves. It might not be enough to cause pain, headaches, or other symptoms, but I wouldn't want the least amount of pressure on my nervous system, and that is why I visit my chiropractor every week. Why every week? I realize that all the different stresses that come into my life every day put more and more pressure on my nervous system, and I always want my master control center working as well as it possibly can. I am not going to wait until my body breaks down to go visit my chiropractor. I would rather take a proactive attitude and get my nervous system and spine checked for interference on a weekly basis. I believe this is one of the main reasons why I feel and look much younger than I actually am, and will continue to hold my weekly visit with my chiropractor for as long as I live.

If you are not sure of all the different stresses that affect your nervous system, this is how I explain the concept to my patients. I usually break stresses down into three different categories. Physical, mental, and chemical stresses bombard us all day long. Examples of physical stresses include working at hard labor, being active with sports, or simply sitting at a desk all day long in one position. Mental stresses can include schoolwork, relationship stresses, or financial worries. We have physical and mental stresses all day long, but the one that really gets us into trouble is chemical stress. We can simply go to the chapter about sugars and completely understand how sugar is a huge toxin and stress on our nervous system. I also usually have my patients list their caffeine intake, prescription drugs, over-the-counter drugs, artificial sweeteners in their diets, etc. Let's not forget about the toxins in the air and water that we take in every day. What about our body-care products such as deodorant, toothpaste and other lotions that we rub into our skin every day? These products that come in contact with our bodies on a daily basis all have toxins in them as well. All of these chemical stresses eventually take a toll on our bodies just as our physical and emotional stresses do. When new patients tell me they have no stresses in their lives, I can't help but laugh.

Day in and day out, all of these stresses take their toll on the nervous system and suppress it little by little. The main purpose of chiropractic is to release that stress from the nervous system and let the body function the way it is supposed to. With the nervous system not working up to par, the body cannot function properly. I have had many patients tell me that as they started their chiropractic care, they noticed they did not get the colds or flu that they were prone to. Others who initially came to my office for back pain would report that not only was their back pain gone, they no longer had acid reflux and did not need to take their heartburn medications anymore. It always puts a smile on my face when patients report these types of results. I never take the praise for great results; I always tell the patient that it's his or her own body that has done the healing. We just helped detoxify, or remove the stress, from the nervous system and the body healed itself and started to function properly. It is amazing how great we can feel when our nervous system is functioning properly.

Your chiropractor should probably be the head of your very own wellness team. Chiropractic is leading the wellness revolution that is taking place, and the nervous system is the most important system of the body, and should be the first system taken care of when starting to *detoxify your life*. Chiropractors have the knowledge, education, and expertise to treat the body as a whole, and many chiropractors now have other wellness experts in their offices with them or have a referral network of other wellness leaders they can quickly and easily refer you to.

Clinical Nutritionist

Since *detoxifying your lifestyle* has a lot to do with what we are putting into our mouths, a clinical nutritionist should be number two on our wellness team hierarchy. A clinical nutritionist is usually a health care provider in some capacity, who has a very thorough understanding of biochemistry and how that relates to anatomy and physiology. The nutritionist will conduct an entire physical examination, testing such things as your skin, hair, saliva, and blood, and performing other specialized tests such as body index analysis (BIA). After the nutritionist gets a good look at your current state, he or she will be able to see what nutrients you are deficient in and what changes you need to make. On your way to *detoxifying your lifestyle*, it is very easy to start eliminating all the junk in your life, but as you start to get the results you want, it is also very easy to fall of the wagon. Regular visits with a clinical nutritionist will help you stay focused and detoxified.

You want to find a nutritionist who is very knowledgeable and has the level of experience and success that you desire. As with the rest of your wellness team, you want to make sure he or she is someone you feel comfortable with, as well as someone who motivates you and brings your energy levels up every time you meet. Many chiropractors have now taken their specialization to nutrition and can do all the lab tests that need to be done, and will be able to suggest a lifestyle-diet program for you as well as high-grade nutritional supplements if needed. Either way, your chiropractor and nutritionist should be working hand in hand with each other and the rest of your wellness team to achieve the best results possible in your health, wellness, and longevity.

Wellness/Life Coach

Let's face it, we all need coaches in our life. Coaches aren't just for athletic teams. All successful people have coaches in their lives. In fact, many have more than one. For example, some of my personal coaches are my financial advisor, my personal trainer, and my golf coach. I also have a business coach and a health and wellness coach as well. My definition of a coach is someone who motivates, teaches, and gives an outlet to reach the goals that have been set forth.

A wellness or life coach could be anyone from your chiropractor to your pastor. It should be someone you meet with on a regular basis to talk to about your life's goals, your current attitudes, your struggles and your accomplishments. You should be able to bounce ideas off your coach and accept his or her constructive criticism.

Wellness and life coaches used to be very rare and very expensive. There are now many coaching programs out there that are very affordable. Usually you will meet or call your coach every week or every other week at a set time to go over your goals and how you are attaining them. You will reach those goals much faster and realize your dreams much more quickly than you would without a coach.

I remember when I hired my first coach. It took me a long time before I actually committed to hiring one. I researched a few and finally made the plunge and hired my very first coach. With that hiring, I personally made a huge mistake by thinking that I no longer needed to work hard because I just paid this coach to do all the work for me. I couldn't have been more wrong, and a lot of individuals make this mistake. A personal coach is not there to do the work for you. He or she is there to simply coach you in the right direction, so you don't make the mistakes that many others have made before you.

Sometimes we get in the mind-set that we can do everything by ourselves, but we need to realize that others came before us, and we should learn from them. That is where coaching comes into play. Their guidance will make our lives much easier and much more rewarding. It will be hard to commit to a wellness coach in the beginning, but once you commit to it, you will be asking yourself why you didn't get a coach much earlier in your life.

A wellness or life coach will keep you motivated and on the right path toward the health and longevity that you deserve. The coach will be able to suggest reading materials that will help you make better decisions with your detoxification process. He or she will give you cutting-edge research with regard to health and wellness, and be there for you when you fall off the wagon to help you get right back up to make better decisions. If you are serious about leading the type of life that you deserve, a wellness coach is someone who will tremendously benefit your family and you.

Personal Trainer

Personal trainers are a dime a dozen. Every gym and health club has them. Sometimes we feel as if they are hounding us. How are we supposed to know who is good for us and who is not? The best thing to do is interview them after reading this book. The chapter on exercise will give you a very adequate knowledge on what type of exercise program you need to lead for longevity. If your trainer doesn't agree with some of the concepts, maybe he or she hasn't kept up with the latest research. So do your due diligence, and make sure your trainer is on the same page as you are.

If you are already an avid exerciser, and are doing the right types of exercise on your own, you might ask yourself if you really need a personal trainer. Well, a trainer isn't someone you have to work out with every single day—although some people need this, especially in the beginning. Maybe you could meet with your trainer just once a month for a workout, and then you can work out by yourself the other twenty-nine days. Do meet with your trainer regularly though, so he or she can test and gauge your progress and tweak your workout regimen for the upcoming month. We never want to get into a rut with our exercise regimen. Trainers are also here to help motivate our workouts and push us to the next level. With that said, definitely add a personal trainer to your wellness team and do meet with him or her regularly for evaluations, updates, and motivation.

Massage Therapist

Massages are great, we all love them. We probably all agree that we do not get them as often as we would like. I believe that massages play a vital role in the detoxification process. Yes, they are a "feel-good" thing or something we do only when it's a special occasion and we want to pamper ourselves, but massages have many health and wellness benefits as well. By living the wellness lifestyle, massages should be a regular habit that we partake in not only because it feels absolutely great, but because it helps rid the body of toxins.

Massage therapists work strictly with the soft tissues of the body. These include our muscles, tendons, and ligaments. With all the stresses and toxins that build up in the body, this is a great way to aid the body in its toxin elimination process. Not only will massage help out with sore, tight, and painful muscles, it will also help relax you and lower your blood pressure. In the relaxation process, you will find yourself breathing more deeply. Throughout your weekly grind of work, getting the kids around, cooking dinner, etc., your stress and tension levels elevate, which speeds up your breathing to rapid, shallow breaths. This isn't particularly good for the long run. Getting a regular massage once a week will help bring your tension levels back to balance. Think of this as your own personal hour every week. No disruptions, no phone calls, no kids to worry about. You deserve at least one hour to yourself each week! I would also recommend you do this midweek; it will give you something to look forward to, and also help you get through the rest of the week.

Another big component of regular massages is the stimulation of the lymphatic system. As we talked about earlier, the lymphatic system is sort of like your body's waste management system. All of your toxins get filtered through the lymphatic vessels, and then eliminated from your body. Massage is a great way to keep your body's waste management system running properly.

Most chiropractic physicians have massage therapists on staff. If yours does not, it is not hard to find one. Check with your local spa or fitness center. You can also ask your personal trainer whom he or she recommends.

Find someone you feel comfortable with and give that massage therapist a try. Do not be afraid to tell your massage therapist what you like or dislike about his or her massaging technique. Some people like fairly deep massages, while others like gentle massages. Find a massage therapist who suits your needs. I can guarantee when you are finished with your massage, you are going to feel relaxed and rejuvenated all at the same time. This is just another vital component that will help you reach your goals of health, wellness, and longevity.

Yoga/Pilates Instructor

We can also clump a lot of other instructors into this category such as an aerobic instructor, Jazzercise instructor, spinning instructor, Tai Chi instructor, and other forms of martial arts as well. We will usually find these types of instructors at our local gyms and health clubs, although many have their own facilities as well. These are people who are very experienced in their own right. They have probably been doing this form of exercise for many years, and have the tools that will help you succeed. They are people who live the wellness lifestyle themselves, and will also keep you motivated during your journey. As we said in the last chapter, we always want to be mixing up a routine and challenging ourselves, so by all means do not be afraid to attend different classes on a weekly basis. Use your instructors by asking questions, and let them know that you want to be challenged to the next level of health, wellness, and longevity.

Naturopath

Naturopathic practitioners concentrate on a holistic approach to wellness. They do not use drugs and surgery for illnesses and disease; instead they use natural remedies such as whole foods and herbs in order to treat dysfunction. They have a certain level of education and are trained to use diagnostic tests to help evaluate the patient. Most naturopaths also focus on detoxification of the organs, and this is why I really like them. Most naturopaths have the same philosophies and beliefs as I do; they believe that healing should start with strengthening and bringing nutrients to the body instead of trying to kill off a certain disease. It is basically Western medicine vs. Eastern medicine. Let's treat the body as a whole and make it as strong as possible before doing anything else.

There are many different kinds of naturopaths with all different kinds of techniques, ideas, and philosophies on healing. Some of the most common techniques that naturopaths use are nutrition, hydrotherapy, different types of manipulation, specific herbs for specific conditions, and different techniques of detoxification. Some believe in a whole body detoxification, while others believe in very specific detoxification, such as a liver detoxification protocol.

I believe in contacting a local naturopath at least a couple of times a year. If you are already making good decisions with your health, you will not have any conditions or diseases that you have to battle with, but it is always good to do a whole body cleanse/ detox at least every six months. A naturopath practitioner will help you find a detoxification protocol that is specific for your needs.

Midwife

A midwife, of course, will need to be part of your team only at a certain point in your life. When you and your partner are planning on having children, you should definitely contact a midwife group to get a basic understanding of what it means to have a natural pregnancy and natural birth.

Midwives, for the most part, believe in a more natural and holistic approach to the entire pregnancy process. From beginning to end, midwives will be there the entire way. They will give you the information needed to take control of your own health as well as your soon-to-be baby's health. They will guide you on different topics such as the right foods to be eating during the different stages of pregnancy as well as different nutritional supplementation that might be needed. The may also offer advice as to specific types of exercises and stretching that need to be done to aid in the process. Midwives will not only be able to guide you throughout the nine months of pregnancy, but they will also be there during the labor process. Some people opt for a home birth, in which the midwife actually delivers the baby. Others feel more comfortable having the baby in a hospital, but still having the midwife present to coach them through the labor process. After pregnancy, most midwives still coach you for the next few months on the proper way to raise the newborn. Again, they will have a much more natural and holistic approach to the entire process, which is much safer for everyone involved.

In practice, midwives refer their clients to me quite regularly. I have noticed that expecting moms that are under the supervision of a midwife have a much more positive outlook on the pregnancy. Coupled with chiropractic care throughout the process, most of these expecting moms have a much easier time as far as morning sickness, back and neck pain, and even actual labor time. It has been my experience that moms under chiropractic care have a much easier time with pregnancy than a typical mom going through pregnancy who hasn't been doing the right things for her body throughout the nine months and whose body is misaligned.

When you and your partner are at this stage in your life, definitely research midwifery a little more, and find one locally whom you feel comfortable with. Your chiropractor will probably know a few good ones in your area.

YOU

Probably the most important teammate we can have on our detox team is YOU! You are the one who gets to make all the final decisions. You get to interview the rest of your team and try out new teammates. You get to decide whether you will listen and follow other wellness professionals' guidance. You get to make your goals and follow through with them.

As adults, we all must be accountable for our own health and wellness. For our kids, we need to teach them the right things to do for their own bodies, and make sure they value themselves, so they will make the right decisions on their own. The best way to teach our children is to show by example. If they see us eating fruits, vegetables, and filtered water all day long, they will think that is normal. If they see us popping four prescription drugs in the morning, making a couple of stops at the local fast-food chain, and taking a couple of ibuprofen at night; then they will think this is normal. Show them that we are meant to be healthy, and if we treat our body right, it will be healthy. Teach them to read labels at the grocery store, what foods to buy regularly, and which foods to stay away from. Show them the right ways to exercise and make it a lifelong goal to stay at your ideal weight. Make health, wellness, and longevity a family fun activity every day.

You should be the most important person. If you don't take care of yourself, how can you take care of others? If you do take care of yourself first and foremost, then you will have the health and energy to take care of others and be much more productive in life. You need to have these health and wellness professionals in your life for education, guidance, and motivation. They are here to help you succeed. Every community has professionals like me who have dedicated their lives to helping others. Try to find people who live the lifestyles they preach. Personally, I wouldn't take health advice from a doctor who is two hundred pounds overweight and hasn't visited his or her local gym in a decade. We need health and wellness professionals who are dedicated to continued learning and also live the wellness lifestyle themselves. If your health provider doesn't even know where the local health market is, maybe you should try to find another professional who is more in line with your wellness philosophies. As you get to the level of health you desire, then you can start helping others out as well. As far as health goes in this country, we are in an uphill battle. My goal is to change one person at a time, and soon have enough people out there talking the wellness lifestyle, and have a snowball effect from there. Be the leader you can be and put your detox team in place to get the results you deserve.

Detoxify Your Lifestyle Today

1. Find a wellness chiropractic clinic to be a part of!!

2. Sign up for a regimen of regular wellness chiropractic adjustments in order to keep your nervous system running properly.

3. Start getting regular wellness massages.

4. Find exercise classes that really challenge you.

5. Find a clinical nutritionist you can seek regular advice from.

6. Find a family physician who leads and preaches a wellness lifestyle.

7. Read one self-help book each month!!

8. Recommit to putting positive people around you and get rid of the negative people.

9. Find an acupuncturist in your area.

10. Be the leader you can be for yourself and your family!!

Your Wellness Care Professionals

<u>Chiropractor:</u> _____
Address _____
Phone # _____
Web site _____

<u>Clinical Nutritionist:</u> _____
Address _____
Phone # _____
Web site _____

<u>Wellness/Life Coach:</u> _____
Address _____
Phone # _____
Web site _____

<u>Personal Trainer:</u> _____
Address _____
Phone # _____
Web site _____

<u>Massage Therapist</u>: _____

Address _____

Phone # _____

Web site _____

<u>Yoga/Pilates Instructor</u>: _____

Address _____

Phone # _____

Web site _____

<u>Naturopath</u>: _____

Address _____

Phone # _____

Web site _____

<u>Midwife</u>: _____

Address _____

Phone # _____

Web site _____

Finally Detoxified

You have officially learned how to *detoxify your lifestyle*. Now it is up to you to take the steps necessary to get the quality of life that you and every other human walking this planet deserve. Through the questionnaires, you should have gauged exactly where you are and how much work you need. Remember, it is not going to be easy by any means, but it is well worth the effort. We all fall off the wagon every so often, but all you have to do is make your next choice a better choice. We have learned that toxins surround us in this day and age. Not that every little toxin affects you drastically, but when we add up all the toxins together, it takes a serious toll on your health and longevity. How good do you want to feel when you are one hundred years old? Do you want to be laying in a nursing home while your caregiver shoves pills down your throat every two hours? Do you want to be able to remember and enjoy your grandchildren and great-grandchildren? Do you want an artificial hip, two artificial knees, a pacemaker, and a couple of artificial valves in your heart at this point in your life? Maybe you would like to be golfing on your 105th birthday. How about going for a swim in the ocean at this age? Maybe you would like to hike through the Rocky Mountains, or simply being able to attend your great-grandchild's college graduation at this age. It is your dream, and I never want to get in between anyone and his or her dreams. I just want to make sure you are able to reach those dreams and goals in this lifetime.

You need to take very seriously everything you have learned in this book. Start applying the wellness attitudes and lifestyles today. Not tomorrow. Go clean out your refrigerator and kitchen cabinets today. Don't wait until next week. The time is now to turn your life around. Go out and get a gym membership today. Go buy your workout shoes today, do not put it off another day. Promise yourself that you will eat out only one meal per week. Learn how to be a better shopper and start reading labels today. Teach your children these wellness beliefs and habits that you have learned and lead our next generation by example.

Maybe you already live the wellness lifestyle. We can always tweak a few things to make it that much better, or add a new exercise program that is more congruent with what your body is meant to do. Maybe you just need to add in some relaxation techniques every morning. Whatever you need, start adding those things into your lifestyle today. You made it this far through *Detoxify Your Lifestyle*, there is no doubt in my mind you can start making positive choices today.

You need to really examine with a microscope everything you put into your mouth, rub on your body, wash your hands with, and everything else that comes into contact with you. Learn how to read labels. You now know that sugar is the most detrimental toxin that you need to be concerned with when shopping for groceries. You should be very motivated to start buying organic produce and meats in order to decrease the toxins in your food.

Once you get started, it is very easy to keep the ball rolling. Pretty soon you will be feeling so good, and full of so much energy that you are not going to believe how you used to live. So many Americans are used to having no energy, being sick with a cold, dragging their feet midday at work, can't get up in the morning, etc. We are so used to feeling like this and thinking it is normal. Trust me—it is not normal. I wish everyone could feel like I do every single morning. Full of energy and ready to conquer the world. You will love the feeling so much that you will start to be contagious and your loved ones will want to start living the wellness lifestyle with you. There is nothing that makes me happier than when I turn an entire family on to the wellness lifestyle. It usually starts with the mother of the household, but the rest of the family soon follows. My number one goal is to turn this entire nation on to wellness. That means a nation without drugs and surgeries. A nation without depression, anxiety, and anger. A nation filled with enjoyment and happiness. A nation filled with energy and motivation. A nation filled with successful people attaining their dreams, goals, and reaching new heights. A nation of families that embrace wellness together. A nation filled with organic-health restaurants instead of fast food. A nation filled with gyms and health clubs that are at full capacity. It starts with us, one at a time. Do it for yourself in the beginning, and then help others get on board with unlimited health, wellness, and longevity.

I wish you luck in your journey to health. Remember that we have only one life to live. Remember that life is the most beautiful thing in the world. Take advantage of it, embrace it, enjoy it, and make it the very best life possible through *detoxifying your lifestyle*. Very good things will soon follow. The only reason that I know what I know today about health, wellness, and longevity is because I refuse to quit learning. I refuse to take Western medicine as the only answer. I urge you to keep reading and learning about the wellness lifestyle. When you are not sure about something, just ask yourself if your ancestors did this, or ate that. It is not the only answer or the only question, but it gives you a good start. I believe I have found a better way to live and I am enjoying every second of it. Jump on board and you will love it as well.

Detoxify Your Lifestyle Now

YOU

1. Stay Motivated and keep learning.
2. Clean out your kitchen.
3. Eliminate sugars from your diet.
4. Eat the right types of fats.
5. Supplement with probiotics.
6. Eat more raw fruits and vegetables.
7. Learn new techniques to cope with your stresses.
8. Start a very specific exercise program.
9. Use wellness professionals to help reach your goals.
10. Share this new knowledge with a loved one.

1. Eric Plasker, *The 100 Year Lifestyle* (Avon, MA: Adams Media, 2007), 5.

2. Marco Studer, M.D. etal., "Effect of Different Antilipidemic Agents and Diets on Mortality," *Archive of Internal Medicine* (2005): 165:725–730.

3. J.N. Din et al. "Omega-3 Fatty Acids and Cardiovascular Disease—Fishing for a Natural Treatment," *British Medical Journal* 328 (2004): 30–35.

4. http://www.whfoods.com/genpage.php?tname=nutrient&dbid=84

5. Eric Ponnanpalam, et al. "Effect of feeding systems on omega-3 fatty acids, conjugated linoleic acid and trans fatty acids in Australian beef cuts:potential impact on human health," Asia Pacific Journal of Clinical Nutrition 15(1) (2006): 21-9.

6. Htttp://www.level1diet.com/fructose-insulin-resistance.html

7. DA Lawlor, "Association of Insulin Resistance with Depression," *British Medical Journal*, 2003 December 13; 327(7428): 1383-1384

8. http://www.mercola.com

9. Nuno Arantes-Oliverira et al. "Healthy Animals with Extreme Longevity" 14 July 2003; accepted 5 September 203, 10.1126/*Science*, 1089169.

10. http://www.ewg.org/sites/foodnews/release.php

11. http://en.wikipedia.org/wiki/Genetically_Modified_Organism

12. http://www.seedsofdeception.com

13. Marwick, C. "Learning how phytochemicals help fight disease." *JAMA*. 1995;274: 1328–1330. Nov 1, 1995

14. Washington Post February 27, 2001; Page HE10

15. C. Ebbeling, et al., "Childhood Obesity," *Lancet;* 360:473-482.

16. Fowler, et al., "New analysis suggests 'diet soda paradox' – less sugar, more weight." *University of Texas Health Science Center at San Antonio. 2005.*

17. Shinichi Kuriyama, MD, et al., "Green Tea Consumption and Mortality Due to Cardiovascular Disease, Cancer, and All Causes in Japan." *JAMA*. 2006;296:1255-1265.

18. K.E. Evers, et al, "A Randomized Clinical Trial of a Population- and Transtheoretical Model-Based Stress-Management Intervention" *Health Psychology* 2002;21:531-541

19. Cordain L, Eaton SB, Miller JB, et. al. "The paradoxical nature of hunter-gatherer diets: meat-based, yet non-atherogenic." *European Journal Clinical Nutriton*. March 2002;56 Suppl 1:S42–52

20. Tomas G. Neilan, MD, et al, "Myocardial Injury and Ventricular Dysfunction Related to Training Levels Among Nonelite Participants in the Boston Marathon"*Circulation*. 2006;114:2325–2333

Author Biography

Dr. Nick Caras is a chiropractor and wellness guru who has helped a number of his patients achieve optimal health through natural remedies rather than the use of drugs and surgery. He currently practices in Denver, Colorado.

Made in the USA